The Fitness Leader's Handbook

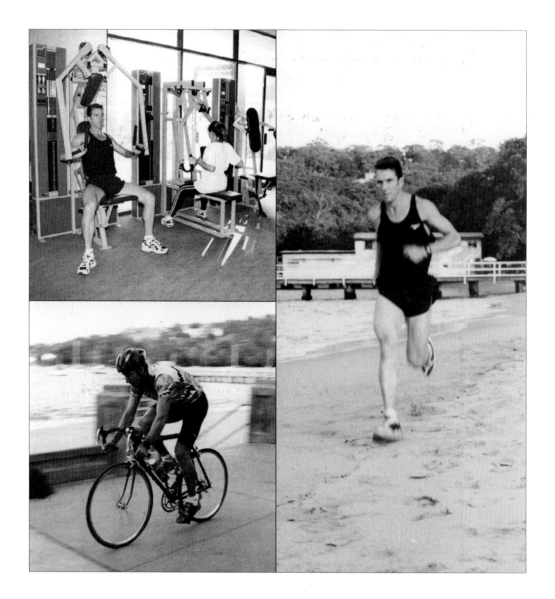

The Fitness Leader's Handbook

FOURTH EDITION

Compiled by
Garry Egger, Nigel Champion and Allan Bolton

A & C Black • London

Contributors

Allan Bolton — BHMS (Hons) Lifestyle Consultant. Director, Productive Personnel Pty. Ltd.

Lisa Champion — MSc Fitness Consultant; Director, Network for Fitness Professionals

Nigel Champion — BPE Director, Network for Fitness Professionals; Convenor ACHPER (NSW) Fitness Leader Training Program

Garry Egger — MPH, PhD Director, Centre for Health Promotion and Research; Adjunct Professor, Deakin University

Cathy Spencer — BAppSc, Fitness Consultant

Rosemary Stanton — BSc, C Nut/Diet, Nutrition Consultant

FISAF

This fourth edition first published in the UK in 1999 by
A & C Black (Publishers) Ltd
37 Soho Square, London W1D 3QZ
www.acblack.com

Reprinted 1999, 2004

Published by special arrangement with
Kangaroo Press, an imprint of Simon & Schuster Australia
20 Barcoo Street, East Roseville NSW 2069

First edition 1983; Second edition 1986; Third edition 1990

Copyright © 1999 by Garry Egger and Nigel Champion

ISBN 0 7136 7029 0

All rights reserved. No part of this publication may be
reproduced in any form or by any means – graphic, electronic
or mechanical, including photocopying, recording, taping or
information storage and retrieval systems – without the
prior permission in writing of the publishers.

A CIP catalogue record for this book
is available from the British Library.

Acknowledgement
Cover photograph © Rick Gomez/CORBIS

Printed and bound in Singapore

Contents

Preface

This book has been written primarily for the training of fitness instructors wishing to gain international certification. It aims to provide all people working, or wishing to work, in the fitness industry with an understanding of the principles for conducting all exercise programs. It has been specifically designed for fitness instructors, teachers, health professionals and others interested in health and fitness.

The first edition of the Fitness Leader's Handbook was written in 1983. Since then the industry internationally has grown rapidly, not only in size, but also in the understanding of scientific exercise principles.

This fourth edition of the Fitness Leader's Handbook outlines the latest research information on potentially dangerous exercises, concisely covers programming principles for weight training, outlines nutritional guidelines in an understandable manner, and provides a scientific basis for the design of safe and effective exercise programs.

We would like to thank the contributing authors for their expertise and co-operation. We are also grateful to all those Fitness Leaders who have given us feedback and advice on how to make this book as applicable as possible to the needs of fitness professionals.

Garry Egger, Nigel Champion and Allan Bolton.

An Introduction
to the Human Body

Knowledge of physical fitness requires a basic understanding of the structure and function of the human body. At the least, this knowledge can help develop a respect for the limitations of the body; it can also aid in planning exercises that are both safe and specific for muscles and joints.

Obviously, such a complex subject can't be covered in a single chapter of a handbook such as this. But it is possible to touch on the basics as they relate to physical activity and exercise.

The Basic Structure of the Body

The basic unit of the body is the cell, which exists in all shapes and sizes. It is within the protoplasm, or jelly-like substance of the cell, that complex biochemical changes occur forming the processes of life as we know it.

Groups of cells combined to perform a similar function are referred to as tissue. Examples are nerves, muscles and connective tissue. These in turn form organs and organ systems such as the heart, lungs, stomach, glands, skeleton and epidermis or skin. Of prime importance to the exerciser are the skeletal system, joints, ligaments, muscles and their attachments, and the cardiorespiratory system.

The Skeletal System

There are 206 bones in the human body, many of which are connected through a variety of joints. If the skeleton consisted of one solid bone, movement would be impossible. To solve this problem nature has developed the skeleton into a system of eleven linked segments, often referred to as the kinetic link system. This link system is divided into two major categories: 1) the axial skeleton which consists of the head, neck, thorax, pelvis and vertebral column and 2) the appendicular skeleton which includes the bones of the upper and lower extremities. These body segments are linked in such a way as to allow movement in multiple directions.

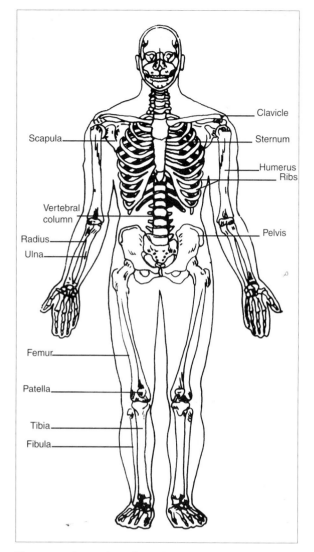

Figure 1.1: **Front view of an adult male human skeleton.**

Labels: Scapula, Clavicle, Sternum, Humerus, Ribs, Vertebral column, Pelvis, Radius, Ulna, Femur, Patella, Tibia, Fibula

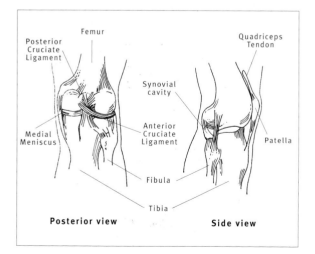

Posterior view   Side view

Labels: Femur, Posterior Cruciate Ligament, Quadriceps Tendon, Synovial cavity, Medial Meniscus, Anterior Cruciate Ligament, Patella, Fibula, Tibia

Figure 1.2: **The structure of a joint (knee joint).**

The skeletal system has five primary functions:

1. **Support** of the soft tissues of the body for maintenance of the body's form and posture.
2. **Movement.** Muscles are attached by tendons to bones which act as levers. When the muscles contract and pull on bones human motion occurs.
3. **Protection.** Bones not linked by moveable joints such as the skull and the rib cage provide protection for important internal organs such as the brain, spinal cord, heart, lungs and the major blood vessels of the thoracic cavity.
4. **Storage** of mineral salts (mostly calcium and phosphorus).
5. **Blood cell production.** In the red marrow of bones red blood cells, some white blood cells and platelets are produced.

Joints are the connections between two or more bones. These can be either fixed (e.g. the ribs) or moveable (e.g. the knee). The moveable joints between bones are those that are used mostly during exercise, and are therefore most prone to misuse, wear and even chronic (gradual) or acute (sudden) injury.

There are five major types of joints, with a basic common structure, shown in Figure 1.2.

The joint cavity between two or more connected bones is surrounded by a **synovial membrane**, within which circulates a jelly-like fluid known as **synovial fluid**. This fluid provides nutrients for the joint surface and lubrication between bone surfaces during movement.

Fibrous bands, called ligaments, connect the bones on the outside of the synovial membrane, giving the joint stability. However, ligaments are relatively inelastic and respond poorly to sudden dislocation of a joint; this often results in permanent damage. It's imperative therefore that correct exercises be prescribed for the various joints so that the ligaments are not overstressed but can develop strength and adaptability.

Within the joint itself, the bone surface is different in structure to the rest of the bone, being both smoother and less dense. This tissue is called the articular cartilage. In addition, some joints (e.g. the knee) have extra pieces of cartilage which help to cushion the impact of the bones.

In the knee joint these cartilages are called menisci.

Major skeletal joints

Ball and socket joints are so called because the ball-like head of one bone fits into the socket of another, permitting circular movements in most directions. Examples are the shoulder and hip joints.

Hinge joints open and shut in a similar fashion to a door hinge. Movements that involve narrowing of the angle between joints are called flexion, and those involving widening of the angle, extension. Movement of typical hinge joints, such as the elbow, knee, jaw, fingers and toes, is limited to flexion and extension.

Vertebral joints connect the large bones of the spine. Each individual joint has only limited movement. However, when the vertebrae move together the spine can bend in all directions as well as rotate.

Sliding joints move from side to side and up and down. They can also rotate, but not as freely as a ball and socket joint. Examples are the wrist and ankle joints, which are also known as ellipsoidal joints.

Pivot joints occur where a ring of bone rotates around a bony prominence on another bone. An example is the first cervical vertebra at the base of the skull which rotates around the second cervical vertebra.

The body as a system of links

The skeletal system is a system of segments linked together at their joints; thus, the body is called a link system. For exercise instructors, the body is best described by eleven links. These are: the head and neck, the thoracic vertebrae, the lumbar vertebrae, the pelvis, the thigh, the lower leg, the foot, the shoulder girdle, the arm, the forearm, and the hands. The movement of the links in the system takes place at the joints of the segments. Each joint is restricted to movement in one, two or three planes of motion — the sagittal (which divides the body into right and left portions), the frontal (front and back), and the transverse (upper and lower).

In order to describe the location of the body systems and the movement terms of these systems it is necessary to have a starting position so that descriptions can be made from a common position. This position is referred to as the anatomical position and requires the subject to stand upright, with the arms by the side (palms facing forwards) and with feet shoulder-width apart. From this postion the following terms are used to describe locations in body structure.

Planes of the body (see Fig. 1.3)

Median is the midline plane dividing the body into left and right halves.

Sagittal is the plane dividing the body into unequal left and right portions. It runs parallel to the median plane.

Frontal (coronal) is the plane dividing the body into unequal front and back parts. The directional terms anterior and posterior relate to this plane.

Transverse (cross-sectional). The transverse plane divides the body into upper (superior) and lower (inferior) parts. Cross or transverse sections are at right angles to the long axis of the body or body segment.

Directions of the body (see Fig. 1.3)

Superior (cranial) refers to a structure being closer to the head or higher than another structure in the body.

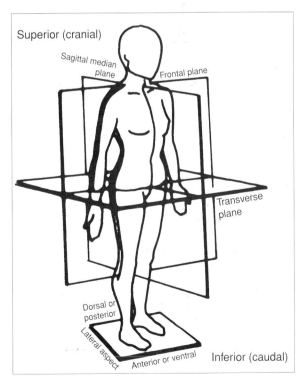

Figure 1.3: **Directions and planes of the body.**

Inferior (caudal) refers to a structure being closer to the feet or lower than another body structure.

Anterior (ventral) refers to a structure that is in front of another body structure in the frontal plane.

Posterior (dorsal) refers to a structure that is behind another body structure in the frontal plane.

Medial refers to a structure being closer to the median plane. For example the tibia is medial to the fibula in the lower leg.

Lateral refers to a structure being further away from the median plane than another structure in the body, e.g. the fibula is lateral to the tibia.

The following two terms are used in reference to the limbs only:

Proximal refers to a structure being closer to the median plane or root of the limb than another structure in the limb. Such a structure is ordinarily superior to the other.

Distal refers to a structure being further from the median plane or root of the limb than another structure in the limb. Such a structure is ordinarily inferior to the other.

Movement terms

The following terms are commonly used to describe movements of the link system.

Flexion: A movement which makes the angle between two bones at their joint smaller than it was when in the anatomical position, e.g. bending the forearm towards the shoulder. Flexion can only occur in the sagittal plane (see Fig. 1.4).

Extension: Opposite action to flexion. It normally involves lengthening of a muscle or widening of the angle between two bones, e.g. straightening the arm in the sagittal plane (see Fig. 1.4).

Hyperextension: Extension beyond the anatomical position.

Abduction: A movement away from the midline of the body, e.g. moving the arms or legs out to the side (see Fig. 1.5).

Adduction: A movement towards the midline of the body, e.g. the arm or the leg that is out to the side of the body being brought towards the midline (see Fig. 1.5).

Circumduction: A movement in a circular direction, e.g. arm circling is circumduction at the shoulder joint.

Pronation: Where, from the anatomical position, the palm of the hand is turned inwards (see Fig. 1.6a).

Supination: Where, from the anatomical position, the palm of the hand is turned outward (see Fig. 1.6a).

Inversion: Rolling of the ankle outwards so the sole is facing towards the midline (see Fig. 1.6b).

Eversion: Rolling of the ankle inwards so the sole is facing outwards or away from the midline (see Fig. 1.6b).

Plantar flexion is where the foot is bent downwards from the ankle, i.e. the toes are pointing down (see Fig. 1.7).

Dorsiflexion is where the foot is bent upwards from the ankle, i.e. the toes are pointing upwards (see Fig. 1.7).

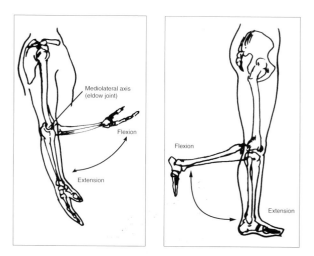

Figure 1.4: **Flexion and extension of the arm and of the leg.**

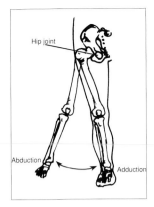

Figure 1.5: **Abduction and adduction of the leg.**

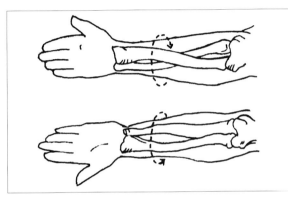

Figure 1.6a: **Pronation and supination of the forearm.**

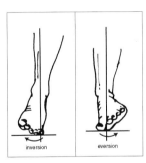

Figure 1.6b: **Eversion and inversion of the foot.**

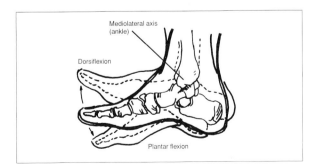

Figure 1.7: **Dorsiflexion and plantar flexion.**

The Muscular System

Approximately 40% of body mass is made up of muscle tissue; the purpose of much of it is to move bones. There are three different types of muscle: smooth muscle (e.g. arteries, stomach), cardiac muscle (i.e. the muscles of the heart) and striated muscle (e.g. arms, legs, etc.). The first two are primarily concerned with involuntary actions. Striated or skeletal muscle, so named because of its striped appearance, generally performs voluntary movements. Skeletal muscle is attached to bone via tendons; on contraction it pulls on the lever system of the body (the bones) and human movement occurs.

There are more than 400 muscles in the body, but those of major importance to the Fitness Leader are shown in Figures 1.8 and 1.9.

There are two important factors that the fitness instructor should consider when studying skeletal muscles for exercise prescription purposes:

1. Skeletal muscles only pull on a bone — they do not push bones.
2. Skeletal muscles usually work in pairs. So, consideration should always be given to training opposing muscles or muscle groups.

Muscles only pull, they do not push

The primary action of skeletal muscles is pulling. Muscles do not push. An example is the biceps muscle, which pulls the forearm to the shoulder. The biceps plays no role in straightening the arm. It is the triceps muscles that pull the arm so that it is straightened to an extended position.

This may appear very simple at first, but when gravity comes into play the whole process becomes more complicated. Take for example the biceps barbell curl exercise. In the upward movement the biceps are shortening while they are contracting (this is known as a concentric or positive contraction) to bring the bar towards the shoulder. As the weight is lowered (the arms are now straightening) the biceps are working against gravity and acting as a braking mechanism. They do this by contracting while the muscle fibres are lengthening (this is known as an eccentric or negative contraction).

Another example is the push-up. Here, the muscles being worked are the pectorals, the deltoids (anterior)

Muscle	Origin	Insertion	Action	Bone moved
Biceps	Shoulder and scapula	Radius	Flexion and supination of forearm	Radius and ulna
Triceps	Humerus and scapula	Ulna	Extension of forearm and extension of shoulder	Radius and ulna
Deltoid	Scapula and clavicle	Humerus	Abduction, flexion and extension of shoulder	Humerus
Trapezius	Base of the skull and C7-T12	Clavicle and scapula	Elevation and adduction of scapula	Scapula
Rhomboids	Spine C7-T5	Scapula	Adduction and downward rotation of scapula	Shoulders
Pectorals	Sternum and clavicle	Humerus	Adduction of humerus and flexion	Humerus
Latissimus doris	Spine T6-L5	Humerus	Extension, rotation and adduction	Humerus
Rectus abdominus	Pubis	Ribs 5, 6 & 7 Xiphoid process	Trunk flexion	
Erector spinae	Lower 7 ribs to L5 and ilium	C1-L5 and ribs	Back extension	
Gluteals	Ilium and sacrum	Femur	Extension and outward rotation	Femur
Quadriceps-Rectus femoris	Ilium	Patella and tibia	Hip flexion and lower leg extension	Femur, tibia and fibula
Hamstrings - Semitendinosus	Ischium	Tibia	Hip extension and lower leg flexion	Femur, tibia and fibula
Gastrocnemius	Femur	Achilles calcaneus	Knee flexion Plantar flexion	Foot
Soleus	Tibia and fibula	Achilles calcaneus	Plantar flexion	Foot
Tibialis anterior	Tibia	Ankle	Dorsiflexion	Foot

Table 1.1: **Muscles and their functions.**

and the triceps. When the body is lowered to the floor the triceps are working eccentrically and when the arms are extended to push up from the floor the triceps are working concentrically. The biceps have no role in the push-up exercise.

Always train the opposing muscle or muscle group

Muscle balance is often a forgotten element in program prescription, whether it be planning an aerobic track or writing a resistance training program. Many of the skeletal muscles work in pairs and if one muscle is overworked at the expense of the opposing muscle it may predispose the area to injury. A common example of this is anterior lower leg pain that is often referred to as 'shin splints'. This complaint can often be attributed to an imbalance between the strong calf muscles (gastrocnemius and soleus) and the weaker muscle in the shin (tibialis anterior). In a floor class the calf muscles

tend to be excessively overloaded due to the amount of jumping exercises and the repetitive foot strike movements that are part of many aerobic tracks. The calf muscles can become overdeveloped and tighten, thereby creating an imbalance with the weaker tibialis anterior muscle. Figure 1.10 lists those muscles that fitness instructors should consider in order to prevent muscle imbalance.

The origin and insertion of skeletal muscles

Each skeletal muscle (i.e. that attached to a bone or bones) has an origin and an insertion and the location of these determines the direction in which it moves a particular bone.

The origin of a muscle is the fixed end or the end which does not move during muscular contraction. The insertion is the attachment at the bone that is moved by the muscle (see Fig. 1.11).

Where a muscle approaches its attachment site with a bone, the contractile elements of that muscle end and connective tissue known as tendons form the attachment. Some of the fibres (called collagen fibres) join with the outside layer of the bone (the periosteum) to form a unit that gives strong resistance to any force against the muscle.

Muscles can either contract (shorten) or relax (lengthen). To move a bone, one or more muscles (called the agonists) contract, while others (called the antagonists) relax, to facilitate the movement. Effective movement of a part of the body therefore depends both on the strength of the agonist, and effective coordination with the antagonist.

The prescription of exercise is highly dependent on the structure and function of the muscle being exercised, and the purpose for which it is being exercised (i.e. strength, flexibility, endurance). Knowledge of the

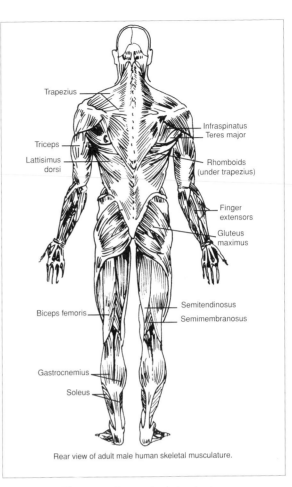

Rear view of adult male human skeletal musculature.

Figure 1.9: **The muscular system: back view.**

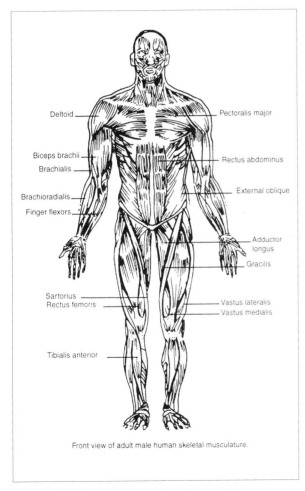

Front view of adult male human skeletal musculature.

Figure 1.8: **The muscular system: front view.**

origins and insertions of a muscle can help identify whether a specific exercise is having the desired effect on a particular muscle.

For example, the traditional method of teaching sit-ups was to instruct the exerciser to keep his or her legs straight, often by hooking the toes under a fixed attachment. However, in this position two groups of muscles come into play — the abdominals (the desired muscle group) and a muscle called the iliopsoas. This muscle has its origin in the bones of the pelvis and spine, and its insertion in the femur (see Fig. 1.12). Because of its connection to the spine, it's thought that if this muscle is selectively over-strengthened, it will cause strain on the lower spine. In any case, it's not the desired muscle for development.

From a knowledge of origins and insertions, it can be reasoned that if the femur is brought towards the spine (i.e. if the leg is bent at the hip), movement of the iliopsoas muscle will be restricted. Bending the knees to

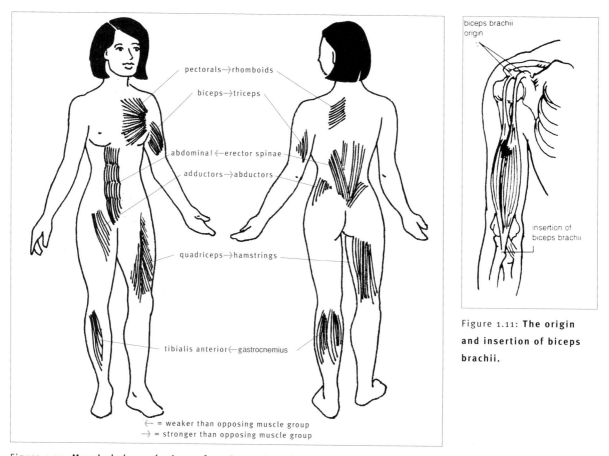

pectorals→rhomboids

biceps→triceps

abdominal←erector spinae

adductors→abductors

quadriceps→hamstrings

tibialis anterior←gastrocnemius

←---- = weaker than opposing muscle group
----→ = stronger than opposing muscle group

biceps brachii
origin

insertion of
biceps brachii

Figure 1.11: **The origin and insertion of biceps brachii.**

Figure 1.10: **Muscle balance (redrawn from Dance Exercise Today, 1988 student handout).**

perform sit-ups then reduces the involvement of the deeper iliopsoas, and increases the involvement of the abdominals. Hence abdominal strengthening through sit-ups should always be carried out with legs bent.

A second example comes from exercises designed to stretch the muscles of the calf. There are two major muscles of interest here: the gastrocnemius or large calf muscle, and the soleus, or deeper calf muscle.

When stretching the calf, as is often advisable before and after activity involving the lower limbs, there are two options. The stretch can be carried out with the leg either straight or bent. With the leg straight, both the soleus and gastrocnemius are stretched. With the leg bent, however, there is no stretching of the gastrocnemius because its origin is above the knee joint. With the knee bent, the distance between its origin and insertion has been shortened to less than the length at which stretching takes place (see Fig. 1.13). The soleus, on the other hand, is stretched much more effectively with the leg bent than with it straight because a greater angle can be achieved at

the ankle joint. Since this is the only joint over which the soleus passes — its origin being below the knee — stretching is maximised through bending the knee.

More detail of muscle physiology in relation to exercise will be covered in Chapter 2.

Overview of muscle contractions and functions

Isometric contractions are where there is no change in the joint angle or muscle length during muscle contraction. It is most representative of an individual's strength production.

Isotonic contractions are where the muscle develops tension while muscle is either shortening or lengthening to move a load. There are two types of isotonic contractions: concentric contractions, where the muscle shortens while contracting, and eccentric contractions where the muscle lengthens while it is contracting (see Chapter 6).

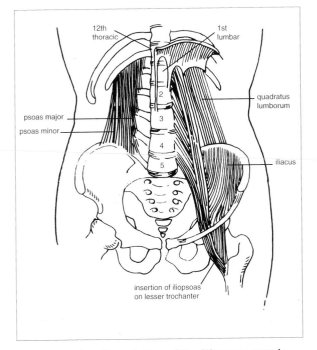

Figure 1.12: **Attachment sites of the iliopsoas muscle.**

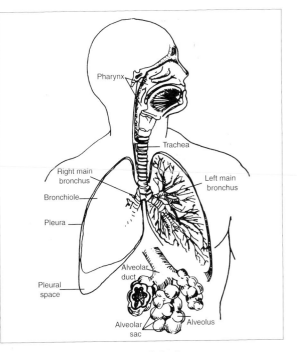

Figure 1.14: **The structures of the lungs.**

Prime movers are muscles that are principally responsible for a given joint movement. For example, in the initial phase of a bench press the pectoralis major is considered the prime mover.

Agonist muscles are those muscles responsible for movement.

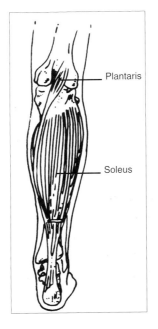

Figure 1.13: **Soleus muscle (shown with overlying gastrocnemius removed).**

Antagonist muscles are the opposing muscles to the agonist (the working muscles); they relax while the agonist contracts. They are not responsible for movement.

Stabilisers are muscles that stabilise one joint so that a desired movement can occur at another joint. For example, during a bicep curl, pectoralis major and latssimus dorsi contract isometrically to stabilise the shoulder joint so that a controlled movement can occur at the elbow joint.

The Cardiorespiratory System

The cardiorespiratory system consists of the cardiovascular system (the heart and blood vessels) and the respiratory system (lungs and air passages). Together, both systems work to transport oxygen from the atmosphere to the cells of the working muscles and organs and to remove carbon dioxide and other waste products.

Blood is the fluid that flows through the circulatory system. Approximately 45% of blood volume is composed of red and white blood cells and blood platelets. The remainder is plasma which carries food, minerals, hormones and chemical substances needed for life. Red blood cells are able to transport and give up oxygen and carbon dioxide through iron-protein molecules called haemoglobin.

The circulatory system consists of vessels called arteries, veins and capillaries, which carry blood from the heart, around the body and return it to the heart.

Arteries have elastic walls to compensate for the surge in pressure each time the heart beats. With the exception of the pulmonary arteries, they transport oxygen-rich blood away from the heart. As the arteries get further from the heart they divide into **arterioles**. These in turn divide again into smaller vessels called capillaries.

Capillaries are microscopic vessels that allow the exchange of oxygen, carbon dioxide, nutrients, hormones and waste products to pass between the blood and the tissues they are servicing. Once the blood has passed through the capillaries it returns to the heart via venuoles that enlarge into veins.

Veins contain valves that ensure that the blood continues to flow in the right direction — towards the heart. The contraction and relaxation of skeletal muscle further assist the return of the blood to the heart. When there is no contraction or relaxation of the muscles, such as when standing in one position for a long period of time, there is a risk of experiencing blood pooling or the accumulation of blood in the large veins in the legs. Fainting can result, leading to a correction of the problem as it removes gravitational effect, enabling the blood to flow back to the heart.

Blood pressure is a measure of the force the heart needs to pump blood through the body. It shows the resistance of the blood vessels to the flow of blood around the circulatory system. Two recordings of blood pressure are taken: systolic and diastolic blood pressure.

Systolic pressure is the pressure on the artery walls when the heart contracts and pumps blood through the body.

Diastolic pressure is the pressure in the artery walls between pumps or heart beats, when the heart is relaxing.

The lungs

The lungs (see Fig. 1.14) are the organs used to exchange air between the blood and the external environment.

Air passes from the environment to the trachea or wind passage and through to the bronchi, which divide into the two lungs. Within each lung, each bronchus divides and subdivides, ending in air sacs called alveoli. It is the alveoli which effect the passage of oxygen into and carbon dioxide out of the blood stream.

At rest, the lungs breathe in about 6 to 8 litres of air per minute. However, this amount increases on exertion resulting in more oxygen being supplied ultimately to the working muscles.

The heart

The heart is a muscle that acts as a pump to circulate blood through the body. It does this at a rate of approximately 72 beats per minute in the average middle-aged male (80 bpm for females), each beat being called a pulse.

The heart, lungs, muscles and organs are connected by veins and arteries that allow blood to be cycled from the lungs, around the body and back again to the lungs for replenishing with oxygen and disposal of wastes (see Fig. 1.15).

The fact that the heart is called upon to supply more blood to an exercising muscle than a resting muscle is important to the Fitness Leader, because it means that pulse rates can be used as a means of determining the individual's response to exercise and an exercise program can be planned accordingly. The workings of the heart and the use of pulse rates will be considered in more detail in Chapters 2 and 4.

Major problems of the cardiovascular system

Coronary artery disease

A heart attack (myocardial infarction) results when an artery carrying blood to the heart muscle (coronary artery) becomes blocked. This generally occurs in the presence of partial blockage caused by a disease called atherosclerosis.

Atherosclerosis is a build-up of fats (cholesterol in particular) and fibrous material on the lining of the

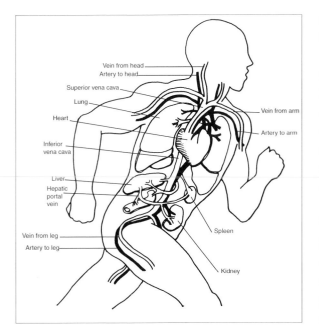

Fig 1.15: **Schematic diagram of circulatory system.**

arteries. This build-up is gradual and takes place over a person's lifetime. When complete blockage occurs, and this is usually a sudden event, a part of the heart muscle loses its blood supply and dies, hence the term myocardial (heart muscle) infarction (death of tissue).

Other cardiac problems associated with atherosclerosis

Angina pectoris is an episode of chest pain or discomfort that may radiate to the neck or jaw, or down either arm to the elbow. It signifies the heart muscle is not receiving sufficient oxygen-rich blood for its immediate needs. Angina usually occurs during physical exertion, emotional arousal or even after a heavy meal where the heart is having to work harder. Angina is not a heart attack but is often considered a precurser to a heart attack. Reducing exercise intensity, or medication in the form of nitroglycerine, usually relieves it. If this is not the case, treat sustained chest pain as a heart attack.

Thrombosis is the blockage of a blood vessel by a blood clot. It is most likely to occur in the presence of atherosclerosis, but also occurs when blood flow is sluggish.

Coronary thrombosis occurs when a clot may block off blood flow to part of the heart, which may cause the affected part to die. If more than 30% of the heart

muscle is damaged death may result. On the other hand, damage to less than 5% may go unnoticed.

Stroke affects the brain — not the heart. It is included here because both stroke and coronary heart disease often share the same underlying causes. A stroke occurs when the blood supply to a part of the brain is either cut off or significantly reduced. When this occurs, part of the brain is starved of oxygen, causing cell damage which may result in paralysis, impaired speech, etc.

Cardiac rehabilitation

Fortunately medical science has progressed to a point where people who have suffered heart disease are not destined to a life of bed rest. In fact cardiac rehabilitation programs are based on getting the patient active as soon as possible. These programs are based on three phases.

Phase I begins when the patient is still in the hospital after suffering a heart attack or after having a cardiac operation. Supervised by a coronary care nurse, small exercise accomplishments are encouraged such as walking down the hall or up a small flight of stairs. During the hospital stay, each exercise accomplishment is recorded and daily increases in the amount of exercise performed are encouraged.

Phase II begins once the patient is released from hospital. They return to the hospital setting three times per week to exercise while being closely monitored. Each person wears mobile ECG leads that transmit back to a monitor watched by the coronary care nurse. Bikes and treadmills are the most common modes of exercise during Phase II. This phase normally lasts for several months. Once the exercise response is stable and the patient feels 'recovered' and passes criteria set by the cardiologist on an exercise ECG test, they graduate on to Phase III.

Phase III is considered a long-term maintenance exercise program. Community facilities or fitness centres are used to provide structured exercise sessions for people who have experienced cardiac events. An exercise specialist trained to work with this population, and a coronary care nurse who is there to help monitor heart rates and blood pressures and to handle any emergencies, supervise the sessions. Emergency medical equipment on site is essential and the program remains affiliated with the hospital.

Valvular disease

The heart has valves which allow blood to flow in one direction but not the other. If these valves become damaged the normal passage of blood flow is interrupted. The damage can often be detected by a heart murmur or a whooshing sound which is clearly audible through a stethoscope.

Arrhythmia

When heart muscle is impaired by an oxygen shortage, the neural stimulation to the cardiac muscle can be affected. This can cause extra heart beats and non-rhythmic muscle contractions that interfere with pumping efficiency.

Arrythmias occur in nearly all people at some time. If they occur spasmodically in individuals without heart problems they are not a cause for concern, but they are causes for concern for individuals with known heart disease.

The Human Body
and Exercise

The human body needs energy to maintain the thousands of processes that sustain life. The term 'energy' describes something that has a capacity to perform work. In the human body, for example, adipose tissue represents a store of chemical energy. Energy occurs in many forms: nuclear, solar, chemical, heat, light, electrical and mechanical. In the biological world all energy originates from the sun, which provides solar energy. The body, however, cannot use solar energy directly; instead it derives chemical energy from food in the form of fats, carbohydrates and proteins. These come from either plants which get their energy from the sun, or animals that eat plants. The energy produced from the breakdown of food is used to synthesise high-energy compounds in the body that are then broken down to release useable energy. These energy-releasing reactions provide the final stage in energy production needed to perform all biological work.

This final stage provides energy for all living tissues in the form of an energy-rich molecule known as adenosine triphosphate (ATP). ATP is the basic energy currency for all biological work (e.g. transmission of nerve impulses,

synthesis of new tissue for growth, repair and reproduction, muscle contraction, etc.). The chemical makeup of ATP is quite complex. The main functional components of ATP, however, are a sugar molecule called adenosine and three phosphate groups (see Fig. 2.1). When ATP is broken down to adenosine diphosphate — ADP (two phosphates) — and a free phosphate molecule, energy is released (Fig 2.1). This energy is used to drive the sliding filament action of muscular contraction explained later in this chapter. In order for the muscle to continue to contract, the ADP must be rebuilt back to ATP. There are a number of processes by which this occurs.

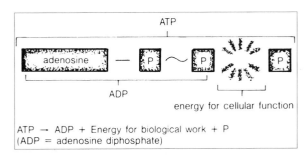

ATP → ADP + Energy for biological work + P
(ADP = adenosine diphosphate)

Figure 2.1: **The ATP molecule.**

The Energy Systems

All human movements require energy and the method by which the body generates energy is determined by the rate of energy demand, that is, the intensity and duration of an activity. Activities that require sudden bursts of effort such as jumping and sprinting need a large production of energy over a short period of time. At the other extreme, activities like distance running and cycling call for continued energy production over a prolonged period at a slower rate.

The first of these types of movement (sudden bursts) are powered by energy systems that don't require oxygen. They're termed anaerobic, which literally means 'without oxygen'. In these cases, energy comes from high-energy phosphate stores in muscle (the phosphate energy system) or via the lactate energy system through anaerobic glycolysis (i.e. the breakdown of glucose without oxygen). This process results in the production of the by-product lactic acid (the lactate energy system). Both of these systems of energy production occur in the cytoplasm of the muscle cell. More extended activities like jogging and cycling require oxygen to produce continued activation of muscles, hence these are called aerobic (with oxygen) activities. Figure 2.2 shows the relationship between the various energy systems.

The aerobic system

The aerobic system is perhaps the most important energy pathway for active individuals to understand because it is the system the body uses for everyday living. It's also the system that predominates in long distance events. In fact, the marathon event is often considered to be a pure aerobic event.

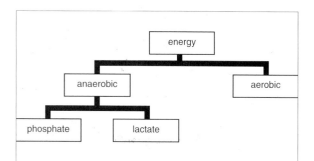

Figure 2.2: **The energy systems.**

The aerobic system is so called because it is energy produced in the presence of sufficient oxygen. As exercise intensity increases the exercising muscles use increasing amounts of oxygen, and glucose becomes the preferred source of fuel, because more energy is derived from the breakdown of glucose per litre of oxygen used. The by-products of the aerobic system are carbon dioxide and water.

As the efficiency of the cardiovascular system in carrying oxygen to the muscles improves through increased fitness, the total amount of oxygen consumed by the working muscles per minute increases. The maximal value, often expressed in terms of millilitres of oxygen per kilogram of bodyweight per minute (ml O_2/kg/min) is called an individual's aerobic capacity or maximal volume of oxygen consumed (MVO_2). Theoretically, a higher MVO_2 indicates an increased ability of the heart to pump blood to the lungs to ventilate oxygen, and of the muscles to take up oxygen.

The series of reactions producing energy via the aerobic system takes place within the muscle cells. But they are confined to specialised sub-cellular sections of muscle tissue called mitochondria. These are often referred to as the 'powerhouses' of the cell because of their role in the aerobic manufacture of ATP.

Aerobic energy production utilises carbohydrates and fats, which are broken down through a series of some 20–25 chemical steps to form ATP with water and carbon dioxide as by-products (see Table 2.1). The water formed is useful within the cell itself and the carbon dioxide is exhaled through the respiratory process. Unlike the anaerobic system, the aerobic system is capable of producing large amounts of ATP without simultaneously generating fatiguing by-products. Basically, activities used to improve aerobic metabolism are those which:

- increase the heart rate (i.e. to >120 beats per minute);
- use 50% or more of total muscle mass, usually including the thighs, trunk, arms and shoulders;
- are carried out over an extended period of at least 20–30 minutes.

Examples include walking, swimming, jogging, cross-country skiing, dancing, cycling, rowing, skipping, circuit training, etc.

Anaerobic energy is simply a way of producing energy without depending on oxygen. This comes into play when the intensity of an activity increases to a point where the cardiorespiratory system can't supply sufficient oxygen to meet the body's energy demands.

The anaerobic system

Anaerobic energy use is like taking money from a bank. If you continue to withdraw without making a deposit you end up in debt. In the same way, an oxygen debt is quickly built up from anaerobic activity that must eventually be repaid: the sprinter has to stop and catch his breath; the footballer has to slow down and jog between explosive sprints.

Within the anaerobic system, there are two distinctly different methods of producing energy: the lactate system and the phosphate system. The former is a means of supplying instant energy through food sources in the absence of oxygen, and the latter comes from the muscles' energy reservoir for instant energy.

The phosphate system

The first process for supplying energy to the muscles is the phosphate system or the ATP-CP system. This comes into play when there is insufficient time for the body to break down glycogen for the manufacture of ATP Although ATP serves as the energy currency for all cells, its quantity is limited, with about 85 grams being stored in the body at any one time. This is enough ATP to sustain about 4–6 seconds of all-out sprint effort. Thus ATP must be constantly re-synthesised to provide a continuous supply of energy. As stored ATP is depleted during sprint-like efforts it is re-synthesised through the breakdown of another high-energy substance stored in muscle

— creatine phosphate (CP). This provides enough energy for 5–10 seconds of maximal effort (see Table 2.1). As rapidly as these energy supplies are broken down, they are restored, to the extent that 50% of the energy source is available 30 seconds later and 100% within 2–5 minutes. As a result, it's possible to repeat many short, intense bouts of activity without becoming exhausted.

In almost all sports, the phosphate system plays a role for short intense bursts of activity. However, if the all-out effort has to continue for longer than about 8–10 seconds, an additional source of energy must be provided for the resynthesis of ATP.

The lactate system

Under circumstances of maximal effort over 10 to 90 seconds, glycogen in the muscles is broken down to form pyruvic acid and then ATP. This process, which is called anaerobic glycolysis, is much less efficient than aerobic glycolysis. It only produces about 5% of the of ATPs produced when glycogen is broken down aerobically. Also, as glycogen is only partially broken down in the absence of oxygen, this results in the formation of a by-product known as lactic acid (see Table 2.1).

If the intensity of the activity is maintained, lactic acid will accumulate in the muscles and blood, resulting in muscle fatigue. Fatigue will start at around 35–40 seconds of vigorous activity, and exhaustion will occur after about 55–60 seconds. Once lactic acid is produced, it requires 45–60 minutes to be removed from the system and for the individual to completely recover.

The lactate system is extremely important as it provides a rapid supply of ATP for intense, short bursts of activity. It also acts as an energy reserve for the middle- or long-distance runner to 'kick' at the finish, or for the

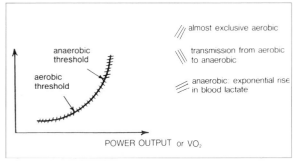

Figure 2.3: **The relationship between aerobic and anaerobic thresholds.**

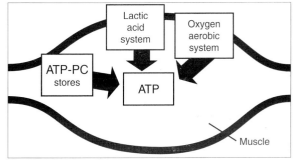

Figure 2.4: **The three systems of energy supply to skeletal muscle.**

	Phosphate (ATP–PC)	Lactic	Aerobic system (with o$_2$)
Energy for muscle contraction			
Anaerobic system (No o$_2$)			
Intensity of effort	Very high intensity 95%–100% of max effort Explosive	High intensity 60%–95% of max effort	Low intensity Up to 70% of max effort
Duration	Only lasts for 10 seconds of explosive activity	60–90 seconds	At low intensity there is no limit
Fuel	Phosphocreatine (PC)	Carbohydrates only In the form of: 1. muscle glycogen 2. blood suger	1. Carbohydrates 2. Fat
By-product	No waste product	Lactic acid	Carbon dioxide (CO_2) — we breathe it out Water (H_2O) — sweat or pass it out
Recovery time	Very quick 50%–30 seconds 100%–2–5 minutes	It takes 20 minutes to 2 hours to break down the lactic acid	Time to replenish glycogen stores up to 48 hrs

Table 2.1: **Energy for muscle contraction.**

footballer to perform repeated bursts of high intensity activity to beat or chase down opponents. Running events ranging from 400 to 800 metres predominantly make use of the lactate system. Middle-distance running on the other hand uses predominantly aerobic energy.

Aerobic/anaerobic Thresholds

Thresholds occur during the progression from low to maximum exercise. The first stage involves primarily aerobic metabolism and is characterised by heart rates below 130 beats per minute and only moderate increases in ventilation. In addition, blood lactate concentrations (a sign of energy intensity) don't change much from resting values.

The second stage, or aerobic threshold, occurs at a point between 40–70% of a person's maximal oxygen uptake (VO$_2$ max). Heart rates rise to 130–150 bpm, ventilation and blood lactate concentration increase, but the effort can be kept up for 3–4 hours. At this level a person can hold a conversation comfortably while exercising.

If the exercise intensity is then increased further past a point where energy cannot be provided fast enough via aerobic metabolism, the anaerobic energy pathway becomes the predominant energy source. This results in a sharp rise in heart rate, blood lactate concentration and ventilation rate (see Fig. 2.3). These physiological responses indicate that an individual is exercising beyond his or her anaerobic threshold (AT) or the point at which lactic acid is produced at too great a rate for the cardiovascular system to process. Other terms used to describe AT are lactate threshold (LT) and the onset of blood lactate accumulation (OBLA). Exercise performed at or above such intensity cannot be maintained for longer than a few minutes.

In endurance athletes the capacity to consume oxygen at or below AT is highly predictive of performance, because exercise performed above AT will quickly lead to fatigue. Hence, given two marathon runners with equal VO$_2$ max measures, the one with a higher AT will perform better as he/she can deliver a greater amount of energy aerobically.

Activity source(s)	Duration	Major energy
Single movement	1 sec.	phosphate
Short sprint	10 sec.	phosphate
Sustained sprint	10–60 secs.	phosphate/lactate
Middle distance sprint	1–6 min.	lactate/aerobic
Marathon	2 hrs+	aerobic
Team games/ extended circuit training, floor classes etc.	1 hour+	phosphate/lactate/ aerobic

Table 2.2: **Examples of different activities and the proportional energy contribution of each energy source.**

The relationship between aerobic and anaerobic energy

Short sprints and sudden bursts of activity are generally anaerobic. General programs for the development of cardiovascular fitness, on the other hand, do not require anaerobic development but should rely primarily on aerobic activities. Most activities and sports call on energy from a combination of the aerobic and anaerobic systems (see Table 2.2).

An intermediate aerobic class utilises a combination of the aerobic and anaerobic energy systems. As such, it is technically incorrect to refer to it simply as an aerobic class. Take for example an intermediate class where the first 35 minutes involves numerous travelling and high/low impact moves. The large muscles of the legs are being predominantly used, requiring a large blood supply. As a result there is an increase in heart rate, which stays elevated for 30 to 35 minutes, thereby overloading the aerobic system. There will be times during this part of the class where the intensity is too great for the aerobic system, resulting in oxygen debt and the subsequent accumulation of lactic acid. In addition the anaerobic (phosphate) pathway may be brought into play during high impact moves that require explosive muscle contractions.

The final part of the class is often structured to overload different muscle groups. Heart rate drops quite significantly as all movements are done more slowly and in a controlled manner. The anaerobic (lactic) pathway becomes the predominant system in this part of the class. Care should be taken to overload the muscles but not to 'burn' them out completely. A newcomer to any extended exercise program, such as an aerobic class, or jogging or swimming, would tire quickly because the aerobic system wouldn't be able to cope with the energy demands placed on it. To overcome this, the body calls on anaerobic sources. But this causes tiredness because of the build-up of lactic acid. As the individual cardiovascularly adapts to the exercise routine the aerobic system becomes more efficient, hence muscles don't have to rely as much on anaerobic sources for energy production. In lay terms, this means the individual is getting 'fitter'.

The energy systems on a run

Another way of looking at the energy continuum is to imagine you are out on a 6 kilometre comfortable run. Energy for jogging along at a comfortable pace comes from the aerobic pathway. Now let's consider when and why the other energy systems may come into play during the run.

While jogging along you come to a reasonably steep hill and you have two choices. The first choice is to slow down and walk up the hill thereby reducing the intensity, which will ensure that you continue to work aerobically. The second choice is to run up the hill at the same speed as when you were running along the flat. If you do this, the intensity of the run is going to be increased significantly. Your heart will have problems supplying the working muscles with the increased oxygen demand, thereby placing you in 'oxygen debt' and causing you to breathe more heavily. In order to service this increase in energy demand, your muscles start to work anaerobically (in the absence of oxygen) and produce the metabolic by-product lactic acid. If the hill is really steep and long you will get into severe oxygen debt and produce large amounts of lactic acid. You may reach a point where your legs start to feel very 'rubbery' and you will have to consider slowing down and maybe even walking. On reaching the top of the hill you cruise down the other side. The heart can easily handle this reduced workload and you start to work aerobically again. The lactic acid is removed from the muscle and broken down by a complex chemical procedure. You are no longer in oxygen debt and can get back to enjoying your run and preparing for the next hill.

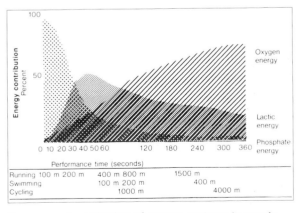

Figure 2.5: **Contribution of energy systems to sports events.**

You have fully recovered from the hill and you are enjoying the scenery when a dog suddenly jumps out of a driveway and starts to chase you. You sprint down the road for 50 metres until the dog loses interest. The energy for this sudden explosive sprint comes from the high energy phosphate stores in your muscles — the ATP-CP system. You only have 8–10 seconds worth of these stored phosphates so if the dog had kept chasing, you might have been in a bit of trouble! With the threat of the dog left behind, you overcome your oxygen debt and slot back into your aerobic system and start to enjoy the scenery again.

Hence, although the ultimate energy currency of muscle contraction is in the form of ATP for jogging along the flat, running up the hill and sprinting from the dog, the means by which it is provided differs according to the type of activity carried out.

The Fuel for Exercise

ATP is made available from the metabolism of food — carbohydrates, proteins and fats. As we have seen, this occurs either aerobically or anaerobically

Carbohydrate as a fuel

The most immediate source of fuel comes from carbohydrates, which are basically sugars and starches. Sugars are the simplest form of carbohydrate. Single unit sugars, known as monosaccharides, are glucose, fructose and galactose. Double sugars or disaccharides are sucrose, lactose and maltose. Sugars tend to be labelled as bad, but in fact they are an important part of the diet. It is the processed sugars that have had all nutritional value removed that should be avoided. Starches are complex carbohydrates known as polysaccharides. They are made up of many units of monosaccharides and are found mainly in cereals, grains, vegetables and legumes. All regularly exercising people should have a diet high in starch and supplemented with sugar. Carbohydrate fuel is stored in the body's cells in two usable forms — glucose (in the blood) and glycogen (in the muscles and liver).

Glucose (often referred to as blood sugar) is the basic usable form of carbohydrate in the body. Blood sugar levels are important to the normal functioning of the

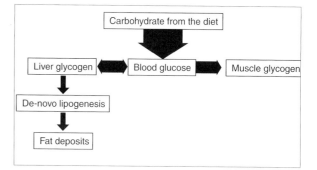

Figure 2.6: **The relationship between carbohydrates, glycogen and fat deposits.**

body, as it is the only fuel that the brain uses. If blood sugar levels are low (hypoglycaemia) lethargy sets in as the whole system starts to slow down. As the name suggests, blood sugar is transported around the body in the blood. In the muscle blood sugar is converted to, and stored as glycogen (a number of glucose molecules linked together). Glycogen is also stored in the liver, which tends to act as the body's reserve tank for carbohydrate. If the body's glycogen stores are full, it is possible for extra energy from glucose to be converted and stored as fat: this process is termed de-novo lipogenesis (see Fig. 2.6.). Some researchers suggest that de-novo lipogenesis only occurs when carbohydrate is over-consumed for about three days at 50% more than daily energy needs. When glycogen is broken down aerobically, it's broken down completely, producing water, CO_2 and energy. On the other hand, when it's broken down anaerobically it's only partially broken down, resulting in the production and accumulation of excess lactic acid.

Fat as a fuel

Like carbohydrate, fat has a basic usable form in the body as free fatty acids (FFA). Triglycerides are the FFAs stored in the adipose (fat) tissue and in the skeletal muscles. The mobilisation of FFA from the fat stores to the muscles is important in the control of body weight, because during prolonged exercise of moderate intensity, FFA represent the major source of fuel for ATP production. Furthermore, FFAs can only be utilised as an energy source via the aerobic system. In practical terms, this means that stored fats are most readily used as fuel during low to moderate intensity activities like moderate walking or jogging, etc. Therefore, for reducing body fat in an overweight, de-conditioned individual, the early stages of an exercise program should be structured around gentle, rhythmic aerobic exercise rather than high intensity anaerobic exercise.

Muscle Physiology

The component of a muscle cell that distinguishes it from all other cells is the myofibril. Skeletal muscle is composed of thousands of these myofibrils bound together by connective tissue and contained in a fluid called sarcoplasm (see Fig. 2.7).

A myofibril contains two basic protein filaments, a thicker one called myosin and a thinner one called actin. It is the arrangement of these filaments that gives a muscle its striped or striated appearance, and it's also the movement of these filaments sliding across each other that causes the muscle to contract (see Fig. 2.8).

The actual mechanism involved in the sliding process is not fully understood. But the suggested process and its connection with ATP production is summarised in the following series of steps:

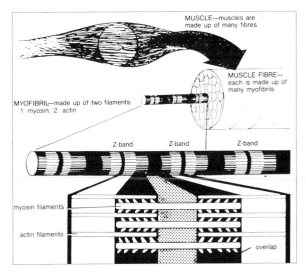

Figure 2.7: **The basic structure of muscle tissue.**

Stage	Muscle action
1. Rest	Cross bridges extended towards actin. Actin and myosin in uncoupled position.
2. Stimulation	Ca++ released. Actin + myosin = actomysin.
3. Contraction	Cross bridges swivel or collapse. Muscle shortens; actin slides over myosin. Tension developed — ATP broken down to ADP + pi + energy.
4. Relaxation	Stimulation ceases. Ca++ removed. Muscle returns to resting state.

Nerves and Muscular Movement

Muscular movement is possible through the stimulation of a muscle via motor nerve, and feedback on the outcome of that movement through the sensory nerves.

The motor unit

The function of the motor nerves is to stimulate the muscle fibres so that they will contract. One motor nerve can service one muscle fibre or several hundred muscle fibres. For example, muscles that perform precise actions like eye movement often have one nerve (motor neuron)

supplying one muscle fibre, whereas in muscles such as the quadriceps, which are responsible for gross actions, a single motor nerve can innervate several hundred muscle fibres. An individual motor nerve fibre plus all the muscle fibres it innervates is called a motor unit. The motor unit is the basic functional entity of muscular activity; it operates according to an all-or-none theory.

An increase in the strength of a muscle can be attributed as much to the number of muscle fibres recruited as to the size of the muscle fibres. For example, if the motor units in the biceps brachii muscle only fire intermittently when doing a biceps curl, the force exerted on the bar is going to be small. On the other hand, if all the motor units fire in unison, then the force generated by the sum total of the muscle fibres recruited will

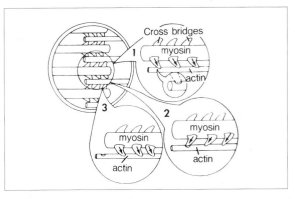

Figure 2.8: **Muscle movement sequence:**
1. **cross bridges extend towards actin;** 2. **cross bridges pull the actin forward;** 3. **stimulation ceases, connection is broken and cross bridges swivel back to next connection, causing muscle to shorten.**

be greater, resulting in a stronger contraction. Recruitment of motor units is based on training stimulus, through which many motor units are taught to fire and contract simultaneously for a given movement. This function of strength is referred to as multiple motor unit summation (number of motor units recruited).

Another function of strength is wave summation, which controls the force produced by one motor unit. Nerves innervate muscle by chemical transmission, which is elicited by an electrical current or nerve impulse. Each impulse (action potential) results in a brief period of muscle activation known as a twitch.

Optimal muscle activation can occur during one twitch, however the nerve impulse is so brief that the muscle relaxes before optimal force production is achieved. Yet, if a second twitch occurs before the muscle relaxes, greater force is achieved through the summation of twitches. Decreasing the time interval between twitches results in greater summation of force. In activities that require precise movement and sensitive adjustments in force application, like handwriting, wave summation is utilised to control pressure.

The most common way of classifying muscle fibres is according to twitch time — fast and slow twitch.

Fast twitch fibres develop force rapidly and have a short twitch time. Time to peak tension = 40 milliseconds (ms).

Slow twitch fibres develop force slowly, consequently having a long twitch time. Time to peak tension = 80–100 ms.

Slow twitch and fast twitch fibres have the same force-generating potential for the same cross-sectional area — but the speed of contraction is different.

The sensory nerves

The function of the sensory nerves (proprioceptors) is to relay to the brain information concerning the tension on muscles, tendons, ligaments and joints. The primary purpose of the proprioceptive system is to make us aware of limb positions and movements in a three-dimensional sense, otherwise referred to as kinesthetic awareness. There are three important proprioceptors that are concerned with kinesthesis: muscle spindles, Golgi tendon organs and joint receptors.

Muscle spindles

Muscle spindles send information to the central nervous system concerning the rate of stretch of a muscle in which they are embedded (see Fig. 2.9). If a muscle is being stretched or lengthened too quickly, the spindle will cause the motor unit to fire and contract that muscle. This prevents the muscle from being overstretched and injured. The slight tightness that is felt whenever a muscle is stretched is the motor nerve stimulating the muscle to contract against the stretch. It is for this reason that bouncy, ballistic or 'double flex' movements are not recommended, especially at the end of the muscle's range of motion.

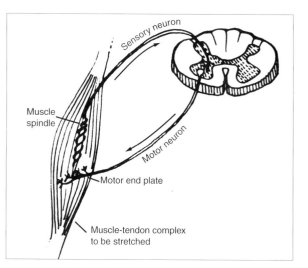

Figure 2.9: **The muscle spindle.**

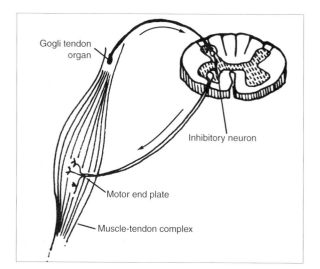

Figure 2.10: **The Golgi tendon organ.**

Golgi tendon organs

These proprioceptors are located near the junction of the muscle and tendon fibres (see Fig. 2.10). The Golgi tendon organs are activated mainly by the force placed upon them by the contraction of the muscles in whose tendons they lie. In contrast to the muscle spindles, stimulation of the Golgi tendon organs results in the inhibition of the muscles in which they are located.

This can be interpreted as a protective function in that during attempts to lift extremely heavy loads that could cause injury, the tendon organs effect a relaxation of the muscles.

It should be pointed out that the spindles and tendon organs work together, the former causing just the right degree of muscular tension to effect a smooth movement and the latter causing muscular relaxation when the load is potentially injurious to the muscles and related structures.

Joint receptors

These receptors are found in tendons, ligaments, bone, muscle and joint capsules. They supply information concerning the joint angle, the acceleration of the joint and the degree of pressure placed on the joint.

All of the above proprioceptors plus other receptors (e.g. sight and sound) are used to give us a sense of awareness of body and limb position, as well as to provide us with automatic reflexes concerned with posture.

Muscle Fibre Types

Two distinct types of muscle fibre have been identified in human skeletal muscle. These are fast twitch (FT) or type II fibres which have high anaerobic capacity, and slow twitch (ST) or type I fibres which have high aerobic capacity.

Fast twitch fibres are characterised by a quick response to a strong stimulus. Physiologically, they have a high capability for anaerobic metabolism, especially in the production of ATP during the initial stages of glycolosis. Athletes in short-term sprint-like activities use predominantly fast twitch fibres, but they are also important in the stop-and-go or change-of-pace sports like basketball or football that require rapid energy from anaerobic pathways.

Slow twitch fibres, on the other hand, have a slower contraction speed than fast twitch. They respond to a lighter stimulus. As might be expected, they become activated in endurance activities, which depend almost entirely on the energy generated by aerobic metabolism. Long-distance running is an example of an activity most suited to slow twitch fibre types. Middle-distance running or swimming, or sports like basketball, hockey and soccer require a blend of both aerobic and anaerobic capacities, and they activate both types of muscle fibres in different proportions (see Table 2.3).

Because of their differences in the use of oxygen, fast and slow twitch muscle fibres generally differ in colour. Slow twitch fibres are darker, usually red in colour, reflecting greater use of the oxygenated blood supply, whereas fast twitch fibres have a whiter appearance.

The differences are obvious in the different muscles of various animals. The legs of a chicken, for example, are dark meat while the wings are white, reflecting the role of the legs in aerobic activity (walking) and of the wings in brief spurts of anaerobic effort (flying).

Fast and slow twitch fibres

As well as ST and FT, two sub-groups of FT fibres have been identified. They are type IIa or fast oxidative glycolytic (FOG) and type IIb or fast glycolytic (FG). The three main types of muscle fibre and their properties are shown in Table 2.4.

Scientists have for a long time been interested in the effects of training on muscle fibre structure. For example, can a sprinter, with a high proportion of FT fibres, increase ST fibres through endurance training? Or can an endurance athlete increase speed potential through intermediate- to high-intensity training?

Activity	% Slow twitch	% Fast twitch	Predominant energy system
Sprint	30	70	phosphate
Middle Distance	60	40	lactate/aerobic
Marathon	80	20	aerobic
Weight Lifting	30	70	phosphate
Hockey	50	50	phosphate/lactate aerobic
Squash	60	40	aerobic/phosphate

Table 2.3: **Percentage of fast and slow twitch fibres in various activities.**

Fibre Type	Metabolic Characteristics	Speed & Strength of Contraction
Slow twitch (ST) Type I Slow oxidative (SO)	High aerobic capacity — low anaerobic capacity — fatigue resistant — red in colour. Small motor nerve.	Slow speed of contraction and low strength of contraction
Fast Twitch (FT) Type IIa Fast oxidative glycolytic (FOG)	Medium aerobic and anaerobic capacity — medium fatigability — whiter in colour. Large motor nerve	Fast speed of contraction and high strength of contraction
Type IIb Fast glycolytic (FG)	Low aerobic capacity — high anaerobic capacity — most fatigable — white in colour. Very large motor nerve	Fast speed of contraction and high strength of contraction

Table 2.4: **Percentage of fast and slow twitch fibres in various activities.**

In general, there are indications that both ST and FT fibres can increase their oxidative (aerobic) capacity through endurance training. It appears that through endurance training Type IIb muscle fibres can become more oxidative and demonstrate Type IIa characteristics. This suggests it may be possible to improve the endurance capacity of a 'sprinter' (i.e. someone with a high FT/ST ratio) through endurance training.

Changes from ST to FT fibres have not occurred in response to sprint training. This implies that the innate 'sprint' ability of an endurance athlete can't be enhanced significantly.

A sudden stop in training may reverse the changes in fibre type produced through training. The ratio of fibre typing appears to be largely genetically determined. However, it appears genetic endowment is of much more importance for sprint type events than for endurance activities.

Despite the classification outlined here, the distinction between fibre types is not clear-cut. There is an overlap of most of the enzymes involved in both major types, and some classifications differentiate between up to 18 different fibre types.

Muscle size

Gains in muscle size usually accompany increases in strength or muscular endurance. The opposite, or atrophy of muscles, results from inactivity.

Increases in muscle size following weight training are thought to be due to an increase in the size of fibres (hypertrophy), rather than the number. However, some research has shown that in some instances the number of fast twitch fibres is increased through a process known as 'longitudinal fibre splitting' or hyperplasia.

Muscle hypertrophy following intensive weight training is thought to be a result of increased fibre size, more total protein, and hypertrophy of connective, tendinous or ligamentous tissues.

Research also indicates that FT fibres respond more to strength training than do ST fibres, by increasing in size. This suggests that the individual suited to power and anaerobic activities (sprinting, throwing, etc.) will tend to bulk more readily in response to resistance training than the individual suited to endurance activity.

Because conversion of fibre types is unlikely (especially from ST to FT), this may imply that the endurance athlete will always have more difficulty adding muscle bulk.

Unlike the opposite, increases in muscle strength do not necessarily mean an increase in muscle size. This is especially so with women, because of the lack of the male hormone testosterone, which influences the development of muscle hypertrophy.

Muscle soreness

Muscle soreness is often attributed to the accumulation of lactic acid in the muscles. This may only be true of acute soreness, where ischaemia, or a decrease in blood flow caused by intense exercise, doesn't allow for the quick removal of metabolic by-products such as lactic acid and potassium.

Delayed soreness usually occurs at least 12 hours after a person performs 'unfamiliar' or vigorous exercise. It can become more severe on the following day and then disappear after some 3–6 days.

The connective tissue theory is perhaps the most scientifically supported theory of muscle pain. This is based on observations that soreness is more common following negative (eccentric) muscle contractions than following positive (concentric) muscle contractions. Research indicates that negative contractions put a greater strain on a muscle's inelastic components (or connective tissue). This is supported by the observation that soreness is usually located in and around the tendon of an eccentrically contracted muscle.

The Cardiorespiratory System and Training

The maintenance of life depends on the efficient operation of the body at the cellular level. Each cell needs a ready supply of oxygen and food, while carbon dioxide and other waste products must be carried away from it.

The heart and the lungs coordinate through the pulmonary circulation system, where de-oxygenated blood is pumped from the right side of the heart (see Fig. 2.11) via the pulmonary arteries to the lungs for oxygenation. (This is the only part of the circulatory system where de-oxygenated blood flows through arteries). Oxygenated blood is then returned to the left side of the heart via the pulmonary veins. (This is the only part of the circulatory system where oxygenated blood flows through veins.) Oxygenated blood is then pumped to the muscles and organs of the body through the systemic circulation system; de-oxygenated blood is returned to the right side of the heart through the veins.

Vigorous exercise increases the need of the muscle cells for oxygen and for removal of waste products. This means that the heart will have to beat faster, resulting in an increase in cardiac output, which increases the blood supply to the working muscle.

If sufficient oxygen does not get through to the muscles, and the intensity of the exercise is maintained, the additional energy requirements will come from the anaerobic system. This results in muscle fatigue through the accumulation of lactic acid. Long-duration activity therefore depends on the ability of the heart and lungs to deliver sufficient oxygen to active muscle.

Cardiac output

To fully meet oxygen demands during exercise two major blood flow changes are necessary:

* An increase in cardiac output (Q), which is the amount of blood pumped by the heart each minute. Cardiac output is measured in litres per minute.
* A redistribution of blood flow from inactive organs to the active muscles.

The increase in cardiac output during exercise is brought about through increases in:

1. Stroke volume: the amount of blood pumped by the left ventricle for each heart beat.
2. Heart rate: the number of times the heart beats per minute.

Mathematically, the relationship of cardiac output (Q) to stroke volume (S.V.) and heart rate (H.R.) is as follows:

Q (litres per minute) = S.V. (litres per beat) x H.R. (beats per min)

For example, if during heavy exercise stroke volume was 0.16 litres per beat and heart rate was 185 beats per minute, cardiac output would be:

Q = 0.16 litre per beat x 185 beats per min = 29.6 litres/min

As a result of an increase in cardiac output the heart will require fewer beats per minute, both during exercise and rest. This improvement in the working capacity of the heart with training, is called a training effect.

Training effect

The human body is a dynamic, responding organism capable of growth and development, atrophy and hypertrophy of tissues. As such, all systems and functions respond to both immediate (exercise) and chronic (training) demands placed upon them. By responding to the immediate elevated demands of exercise, the organs and systems stressed are forced to function at a level above that to which they are normally accustomed. This stimulus, when repeated at regular intervals of

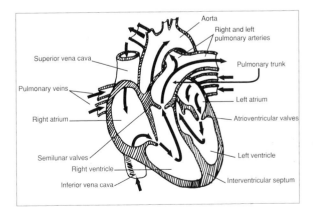

Figure 2.11: **The human heart.**

sufficient frequency, intensity and duration, produces a training effect that enables a higher maximal training function than before.

Venous return

Regardless of the mechanisms that increase cardiac output during exercise, the heart can pump only as much as it receives. For this reason, cardiac output is ultimately dependent on the amount of blood returned to the heart in other words, upon the venous return.

The primary mechanism for increasing the venous return during exercise is the muscle pump. The muscle pump is the result of the mechanical pumping action produced by rhythmical muscular contractions. As the muscles contract, their veins are compressed and the blood within them is forced towards the heart. Blood is prevented from flowing backwards because veins contain numerous valves that permit flow only towards the heart.

If the muscle pump is not working, as is the case when you stand still for a long time or immediately stop following a workout, then blood pooling occurs, resulting in insufficient blood flow to the brain and fainting may result.

Heart rates

While the average pulse rate of a sedentary man is around 72 bpm and of a woman around 80 bpm, these rates are often significantly less in trained athletes. Marathon runners have recorded resting heart rates as low as 30–35 bpm.

Heart rate responses to standard workloads have, over the years, been used as an indication of changes in physical fitness. With training that raises the heart rate (HR) above a standard work load (often estimated from formulae using age-estimated maximal heart rates), the working HR will decrease, enabling a greater work load to be carried out with the same effort. Heart rate, then, is an important feedback mechanism for any exerciser or exercise programmer, as we shall see in Chapter 4.

Blood vessels

During exertion there is a redistribution of blood flow from the organs of the body to the working muscles so that these receive a greater proportion of cardiac output. This redistribution of blood flow is dependent on the vasoconstriction (narrowing) of arterioles supplying the inactive parts of the body, such as the kidneys, liver and stomach, and the vasodilation (opening) of arterioles to the skeletal muscles being used in the activity. With training this whole system becomes more efficient, thereby always supplying skeletal muscles with sufficient blood flow.

Maximal pulse is the highest an individual's heart rate will go. This generally declines with age from around 220 bpm in under-20-year-olds to around 160 bpm in over-60-year-olds.

Blood pressure and exercise

Systolic and diastolic pressure average around 120 mmHg and 80 mmHg respectively with a mean pressure of about 93 mmHg. The mean arterial pressure is the average of the systemic systolic and diastolic pressures during a complete cycle (systole plus diastole).

During exercise, blood pressure increases as a result of the accompanying increase in cardiac output. In fact, exercise affects systolic blood pressure more than diastolic or mean pressure. This is because during exercise there is a simultaneous decrease in resistance as a result of vasodilation of the arterioles supplying blood to the active skeletal muscles. This means that blood will drain from the arteries through the arterioles and into the muscle capillaries, thus minimising changes in diastolic pressure.

Maximal oxygen uptake

Maximal oxygen uptake (VO_2max), is the maximal amount of oxygen capable of being transported to and consumed by the working muscles. In other words, it can be used as a measure of aerobic fitness. At rest, the body uses about 3.5 millilitres of oxygen per kilogram of body weight per minute (3.5 ml/kg/min) to sustain life. Measures of VO_2 max have been recorded as high as 92 ml/kg/min — scores like this are characteristic of elite endurance athletes. A low VO_2max, indicating poor fitness in a middle-aged man, would be around 26 ml/kg/min. Examples of VO_2max recordings are shown in Figure 2.12.

As physical fitness and the capacity of the heart improve with training, oxygen uptake will improve significantly. This can be demonstrated in tests of aerobic capacity.

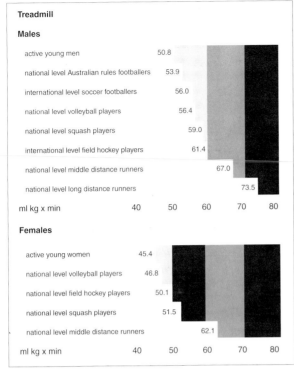

Treadmill

Males

	ml kg x min
active young men	50.8
national level Australian rules footballers	53.9
international level soccer footballers	56.0
national level volleyball players	56.4
national level squash players	59.0
international level field hockey players	61.4
national level middle distance runners	67.0
national level long distance runners	73.5

ml kg x min   40   50   60   70   80

Females

	ml kg x min
active young women	45.4
national level volleyball players	46.8
national level field hockey players	50.1
national level squash players	51.5
national level middle distance runners	62.1

ml kg x min   40   50   60   70   80

Figure 2.12: **Maximal oxygen uptake values obtained on Australian sportsmen and sportswomen.**

Another measure of aerobic capacity is the MET, short for basic metabolic unit. One MET is the amount of oxygen used by the body at rest (i.e. around 3.5 ml/kg/min), and maximal oxygen uptake is expressed in terms of multiples of this unit or max METs. MET scores can be equated with VO_2max scores by multiplying Mets by 10. In training for cardiovascular improvement, exercises at a predetermined MET level (generally 60–80% of max METs) are often used to ensure sufficient individual effort to establish a training effect. A low intensity aerobic class could have an exercise intensity of 8 METs. Expressed as oxygen consumption this will be 8 x 3.5 = 28 ml/kg/min.

Hydration

The body dissipates most of its heat through two primary avenues:

1. Radiation through peripheral vasodilation where warm blood is taken from within the body to the periphery for cooling. The main disadvantage with this avenue of heat loss is that blood is directed away from the working muscles where it is needed, leading to oxygen debt.

2. Evaporation. This refers to the dissipation of heat from the body through the evaporation of sweat. In fact, the sweat that is seen dripping off the body does not cool the body. It is the sweat that is not seen (evaporated) that cools the body. For this reason exercising in a hot, humid environment increases the risk of heat stress due to the amount of water vapour in the atmosphere (see Fig. 2.13).

The evaporation of sweat from the skin is an extremely effective means of dissipating the heat produced during exercise. For this reason, sweating is the most important thermoregulatory response during exercise. The downside is that sweating occurs at the expense of the body's fluid stores. The resulting dehydration impairs physiological function, hampers performance and drastically increases the risk of heat illness.

Well-conditioned athletes who are acclimatised to exercise in the heat can lose immense volumes of sweat. It is not uncommon for athletes to lose in excess of 2 litres of sweat per hour; sweat losses ranging between 1 to 2 litres per hour are commonplace (1 litre of water is equivalent to 1 kilogram of body weight). It has been reported that marathon runners can lose in excess of 6 litres of sweat, even during an event conducted in cool conditions.

A sweat loss equivalent to as little as a 1% decrease in body weight impairs the body's temperature-regulating capacity and increases the stress on the cardiovascular system. As the extent of dehydration increases, these detrimental effects on performance and health also increase. While it is not unusual for athletes to finish a practice or competition dehydrated with a 3% to 4% decrease in body weight, preventing this dehydration will allow them to work longer and harder, ultimately benefiting competitive performance. It is important to note that the dangers of heat disorders and dehydration are not just restricted to the endurance athlete, but to anyone exercising in hot or humid environments.

When the body loses excessive fluid, as can occur with dehydration, the blood becomes more viscous (thicker) and its ability to flow is significantly reduced.

This results in an insufficient blood supply to the working muscles, which consequently lose their ability to work aerobically. At this point either the effort must be reduced, or the muscles generate energy anaerobically, a process which can only be continued for a limited period of time.

Not replacing body fluids after exercise results in a feeling of lethargy and, in some instances, dizziness associated with an elevated heart rate. In some cases, fluid losses are even considered as a (misguided) means of losing weight. Water contains no calories, hence the drinking of fluid will not affect body fat.

The exerciser therefore has to be conscious of how to replace this fluid and what forms this replacement should take. Should one drink plain water or a sports drink? Maintenance of hydration has been the subject of a substantial amount of research recently. This research has focused primarily on five areas:

1. **Effect of beverage palatability and composition on voluntary fluid consumption.** Sports drinks must be formulated to taste best when people are hot and sweaty. Drinks that appeal to people at rest usually do not have the same appeal during exercise. Although the physiological reasons for this change in preference are not well understood, research has shown that athletes prefer non-carbonated, citrus-flavoured drinks that are slightly sweet, have a light mouthfeel and a quickly disappearing aftertaste.

2. **Gastric emptying and intestinal absorption of fluids.** In addition to encouraging voluntary fluid intake, a fluid replacement drink must also facilitate fluid absorption, i.e. a drink that can exit rapidly from the stomach and be quickly absorbed from the small intestine into the bloodstream. Research has found that water and many sports drinks have similar gastric emptying rates during exercise. However, several commercially available sports drinks are absorbed through the small intestine significantly faster than plain water during exercise and at rest. Experts recommend a 6–7% carbohydrate concentration for optimal fluid absorption and energy provision. For this reason, fruit juices, fruit drinks and soft drinks are contraindicated for use during exercise.

3. **Cardiovascular and thermoregulatory responses to fluid ingestion.** Fluid consumption during exercise is vital for two primary purposes — safeguarding health and optimising athletic performance. Research repeatedly demonstrates that dehydration of as little as 1% of body weight can impair the body's ability to regulate temperature, can cause fatigue and reduce performance levels. Cardiovascular and thermoregulatory functions are best maintained when athletes ingest fluid in quantities that closely approximate the volume of sweat loss.

4. **Carbohydrate feeding and exercise performance.** Research from numerous universities around the world has repeatedly shown performance benefits from ingesting carbohydrate during exercise. Consumption of sports drinks containing carbohydrate compared to plain water allows athletes to work longer and harder. Consuming carbohydrate helps maintain blood glucose and increases carbohydrate oxidation, assuring skeletal muscle and the central nervous system an ample supply of energy. Ingesting 25–75 grams of carbohydrate at a suitable concentration each hour is sufficient to spark improvement in exercise performance. Drinking beverages that contain more than 6–7% carbohydrate does not result in a further improvement in exercise performance. It is recommended that sports drinks use a combination of glucose, fructose and maltodextrin as carbohydrate sources. Drinks that use only fructose can cause gastric distress.

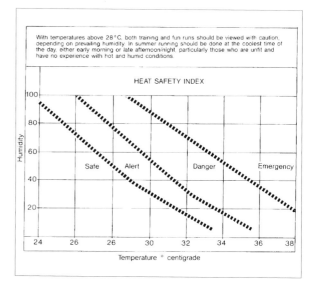

Figure 2.13: **Heat stress index.**

5. **Beverage composition and the rate of rehydration.** The rate at which the body fully rehydrates following exercise depends on the amount and composition of the drink used. Research has shown that rehydration is more complete with certain sports drinks than with water or carbonated soft drinks. Along with glucose, drinks should contain sodium as this stimulates fluid absorption and promotes fluid balance, maintains the desire to drink, enhances taste and helps the body hold on to water — all important factors for rehydration.

Although drinking fluids during exercise is the very best way to prevent dehydration and maintain physiological function, most people finish exercise at least slightly dehydrated. Complete restoration of body fluid balance can occur only when the sodium chloride that was lost in sweat is replaced. This is usually accomplished by eating meals, making rehydration a slow process up to 12 hours. However, there are many occasions when athletes, workers and soldiers must rehydrate quickly. In such cases, consuming properly formulated carbohdrate-electrolyte drink results in the rapid and complete rehydration that cannot be achieved with other fluids.

The sodium and glucose in sports drinks provide an osmotic impetus to maintain thirst and stimulate the rapid restoration of intra and extra-cellular fluid volumes. Drinks that do not contain sodium will be ineffective in assuring complete rehydration.

Other recommendations for maintenance of fluid balance are:

🏃 Drink 2 glasses (300–500 ml) of fluid 15–20 minutes before heavy exercise and one glass (150–250 ml) at 15–20 minute intervals throughout the activity. Continue drinking after exercise.

🏃 If competing in endurance activities (e.g. a marathon), take regular drinks at drink stops from the start. Because it takes time for fluids to pass through the system, these should be ingested before thirst is felt.

🏃 Consider ambient conditions, avoid performing long bouts of exercise in hot, humid conditions. Use the heat stress index shown in Figure 2.13 as a safety guide.

Principles of Exercise Programming

Exercise is a major factor in the maintenance of health of an individual. Among its proven benefits are:

- Increased physical work capacity (strength, endurance).
- Increased cardiovascular and respiratory efficiency.
- Decreased risk of coronary heart disease.
- Changes in body metabolism (e.g. reduced level of obesity).
- Delay of physiological ageing effects.
- Psychological effects (e.g. stress reduction, increased self-confidence).

Exercise programmes can be designed to develop one or a number of aspects of physical fitness. For example, there's fitness for cardiovascular (heart/lung) efficiency, for strength, speed, flexibility, muscle endurance, power, agility and balance.

Each aspect of fitness involves varying contributions of the energy systems discussed in Chapter 2. Which type of fitness is important will depend on the needs of an individual. A shot-putter, for example, will

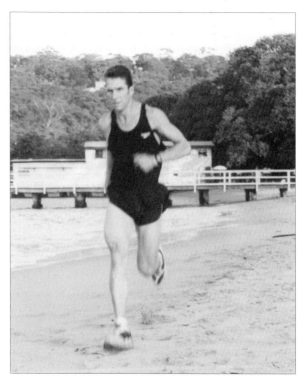

A minimum amount of exercise is required to produce a training effect.

need strength and power but little agility, while a marathon runner would need cardiorespiratory fitness and muscle endurance but not necessarily strength, agility or balance.

Training for specific purposes is covered in more detail in sports training texts. Here we're interested primarily in the types of fitness that will most benefit the non-competing population. In particular these are:

1. Cardiovascular fitness (**Stamina**),
2. Flexibility (**Suppleness**),
3. Muscular strength (**Strength**)
4. **Speed.**

They've been called the **Four S's of Fitness**. We'll look at the first three in the chapters that follow.

Principles of Exercise Prescription

The first step in exercise programming is to establish a specific objective: to determine which physical parameters are to be improved. If reductions in body weight and improved aerobic fitness are important, aerobic exercise will be indicated. If muscle and joint stiffness is a problem, flexibility training should play a large part. If muscle strength is low and needs to be increased, some strengthening work should be included.

Next, a program should be designed to meet the established objectives. This necessarily involves decisions about the type, duration and frequency of exercise as well as the means to evaluate progress in the form of relevant physiological and/or performance tests.

The training threshold

There is a minimum amount of exercise that is required to produce significant improvements in any physical fitness parameter. This is referred to as the training threshold. For example, the recognised training threshold for the development of aerobic fitness in most people is regarded as 20–60 minutes of effort at a heart rate of between 60% and 80% of maximum heart rate or MHR (see Chapter 4).

Overload

The overload principle also applies to all types of training. This implies that an individual must exercise at a level above that which can be normally carried out comfortably. For example, to increase the strength of a muscle, it must be contracted against a greater than normal resistance. The intensity, duration and frequency of exercise, therefore, should be above the training threshold and be gradually but progressively increased as the body adapts to the increasing demands. As fitness levels improve, so the training threshold will be raised (see Chapter 6).

Specificity

The principle of specificity of training effect implies that different forms of exercise produce different results. The type of exercise carried out is specific both to the muscle groups being used and to the energy sources involved. For example, there is little transfer of training from strength training to the cardiovascular system. Similarly, prolonged running is unlikely to improve endurance swimming performances.

This was demonstrated in a study using a group of 20 men who were trained on a bicycle ergometer over an 8-week period and tested before and after on both the bicycle ergometer and a treadmill. Maximal oxygen uptake improved 7.8% as measured by the bicycle ergometer, but only 2.6% as measured on the treadmill. In another study, swimming was used as the primary training technique over 10 weeks and subjects were tested before and after on swimming and running (treadmill) tests. Results showed an improvement of 11% in VO_2 max. as measured by the swimming test, but there was no improvement in the treadmill. Improvements in this case were apparently so specific as to be non-transferable to exercise involving other large muscle groups.

Reversibility

Training effects are reversible in that if workouts stop or are not done often enough or with sufficient intensity, benefits can be lost quickly. Continuing training at a maintenance level after a high level of conditioning has been obtained can prevent loss of benefits.

Progression

As a person becomes fitter, a higher intensity of exercise is required to create an overload and therefore provide continued improvements. This is most pertinent for athletes who wish not merely to maintain a good level of fitness but to improve on that level. Progression can be through either increased intensity or duration of exercise sessions.

Warm-up

Every exercise session should be preceded by a period of warm-up where the body is prepared gradually for the effort to come. Warm-up should be gentle and rhythmic and preferably use the joints and muscles to be involved in the major activity. It should take up 10–20% of the time spent in the primary exercise (see Chapters 4 and 8).

Cool-down

As with the warm-up, a cool-down period is a vital component of an exercise session. This involves a gradual decrease in the intensity of the exercise until the body's physiological functions return to the resting state. An adequate cool-down helps the muscles of the body return blood to the heart rather than pool in the muscles (see Chapters 4 and 8).

Types of exercise programs

In this book we'll be focussing on training programs for three of the four S's — stamina, suppleness and strength. Only a general run-down of each will be given in this chapter. More detailed exercise programs will be covered in Chapters 4, 5 and 6.

Somatotyping

Somatotyping is an effective way of classifying people based on their overall body shape. It is a good technique because it is a classification of total body shape that can be expressed as a single rating. The rating represents the evaluation of body shape following the three components of physique illustrated in Fig. 3.1.

Better Coaching — Advanced Coach's Manual, ed. F.S. Pyke, Australian Coaching Council, 1991 explains that the somatotype rating for a person is given as three successive hyphenated numerals (with a highest rating of 7): e.g. 4–5–3 with the three numerals representing endomorphy, mesomorphy and ectomorphy — always in that order. In general, ratings from 1 to 2 are regarded as low values; ratings of 3 to 5 are regarded as mid range and ratings of 5 are high.

Cardiorespiratory Training (Stamina)

Cardiorespiratory fitness is often called aerobic fitness because it involves predominantly aerobic energy. It is usually regarded as the most important aspect of community fitness because of its relationship to coronary heart disease (CHD) and control of body fat levels.

People who regularly exercise aerobically have a lower incidence of coronary heart disease than those who remain sedentary. In fact, according to Dr Ralph Paffenbarger, Professor of Epidemiology at Stanford University, who has carried out much research into the benefits of exercise:

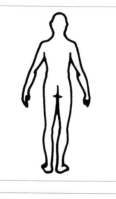

Ectomorph
Refers to the relative linearity of the body.

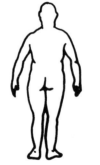

Endomorph
Refers to the relative fatness of the body.

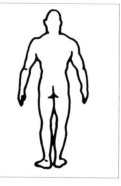

Mesomorph
Refers to the relative muscular development per unit height of the body.

Figure 3.1: **The three basic physique types (*Better Coaching*, ed. F.S. Pyke, ACC 1991)**

'... strenuous and continual exercise provides the greatest protection with the possible exception of lowered blood pressure against death from heart disease.'

Of course any exercise, if not carried out properly, can be dangerous for some people. In cases where heart disease is advanced, for example, sudden excessive exertion may bring on heart failure. Yet the chances of these events occurring in a healthy person are minute. To understand just how much so, we need to look at some statistics.

The dangers of exercise

According to Dr Roy Shephard, Professor of Preventive Medicine at the University of Toronto in Canada, the chances of a normal man having a heart attack during one half-hour session of heavy exercise is 1 in 5 million. In a normal woman, the chance is 1 in 17 million.

The most detailed Australian study of sudden deaths has shown that only 7% were associated with strenuous exercise. The other 93% occurred while the victim was carrying out everyday activities such as standing, sitting still or lying down.

Similarly, Dr Ernst Jokl in his book on *Exercise and Cardiac Death* points out that sudden deaths do not occur in persons with a healthy heart. Says Jokl: 'Not one instance was encountered in which death could be regarded as due to the effects of extreme exertion on a previously healthy heart.'

Exercise does have risks, particularly for the previously sedentary person. But these need to be weighed against the risks of not exercising. Then a decision can be made as to which is the more dangerous path to take.

Developing aerobic fitness

To develop 'aerobic' fitness, it is necessary to exercise at an intensity above the training threshold (generally around 60% of the maximum heart rate) for a period of 15–60 minutes, on 3–5 days each week. Exercise may be continuous such as with LSD (long slow distance) training, or it may be intermittent, where intervals of exercise are interspersed with periods of rest or mild exercise (interval training). Circuit training is another form of aerobic conditioning that also includes aspects of strength and flexibility.

In circuit training, the individual is given a variety of exercises to do continuously. While the exercises in isolation may not be aerobic, when performed continuously in a set sequence they readily become so. Continuous exercise may be more appropriate for individuals with low fitness levels, while intermittent exercise is seen as being superior for preparing an athlete for competitive sports where high-level fitness is important (see Chapter 4).

Aerobic conditioning guidelines

Some basic rules for the development of aerobic fitness are:

- If you don't exercise regularly, are over 35 years of age or have any major health problems (see Chapter 4), have a medical examination before starting an exercise program.
- Warm up gradually at the start of each session and cool down gradually at the end. Stretching exercises (see Chapter 5) should immediately follow the general warm-up session.
- Carry out physical activity involving large muscle groups, e.g. jogging, swimming, cycling, etc.
- Start the program slowly and increase the intensity, duration and frequency of exercises gradually until they conform to prescription.
- Avoid sudden exercise of unaccustomed intensity. Any change of activity should be gradual.
- Wear well-fitting, appropriate shoes if running.
- Use your heart rate as a guide to the intensity of exercise.

More details of aerobic conditioning are covered in Chapter 4.

Flexibility Training (Suppleness)

Flexibility training involves stretching of muscles and tendons to maintain or increase suppleness. Stretching can be of four major types:

1. **Static stretching:** This involves the gradual lengthening of a muscle to a stretched position, where it is held.
2. **PNF stretching:** PNF (proprioceptive neuromuscular facilitation) stretching is a form of static stretching incorporating isometric contraction of the stretched muscle. PNF stretching takes advantage

of the function of the Golgi tendon organ discussed in Chapter 2. When the Golgi tendon organ is stimulated by the force of the muscle contraction, the muscle relaxes and can be stretched through a greater range than normal. PNF stretching is the type now recommended by most sports medicine experts for flexibility and injury rehabilitation.

2. **Range of motion (ROM) stretching:** ROM stretching involves the rhythmical movement of major joints and associated muscle groups that are used in an activity through their full range of movement.

4. **Ballistic stretching:** Often called 'dynamic' stretching, this involves bouncing or movement at a joint's end-range of motion. It is not recommended because it can result in injury due to the stretch reflex (see Chapter 2). If over-stretching through bouncing occurs, the result may be a tightening of the muscle rather than the desired loosening.

A high degree of flexibility is desirable for some activities and a reasonable degree is important for the prevention of soft tissue injuries. An adequate warm-up, which involves large muscle groups and whole body movements, should precede stretching.

Flexibility is highly joint-specific, meaning that a high degree of flexibility in one joint doesn't necessarily mean that the same degree of flexibility will exist in other joints. To improve flexibility, the muscle should be stretched beyond its normal length.

More details on flexibility training are given in Chapter 5.

Muscle Training (Strength)

As we saw in Chapter 2, there are two main types of muscle fibre: fast twitch and slow twitch. Fast twitch fibres are used predominantly in strength and power activities, while slow twitch fibres are used in aerobic exercise. Strength training that uses high resistance usually develops the fast twitch fibres selectively.

Muscular endurance training can also be carried out with weights or resistance. The appropriate regimen is low-resistance exercise repeated many times.

Strength training may be isotonic, isometric, or isokinetic. All three methods have been shown to be effective, but since strength development is highly specific, the nature of the performance to be improved should determine the method adopted.

Isotonic training involves the contraction of a muscle against a moveable resistance (e.g. free weights). Contraction may occur while the muscle is shortening, in which case it is called a concentric (or positive) contraction (e.g. the biceps while raising a weight during elbow flexion). Contraction may also occur while the muscle is lengthening, in which case it is called an eccentric (or negative) contraction (e.g. during elbow extension with the biceps lowering a weight).

Isometric training involves static muscle contractions against an immovable resistance, e.g. pushing against a solid wall.

Isokinetic training involves contraction of muscle at a set rotational speed through a set range of motions. This is based on the principle that a muscle exerts different force at different stages in a contraction. In theory, to work the muscle maximally throughout the contraction requires a continuous monitoring of muscle movement and a variable adjustment of resistance at each stage of the movement.

Exercise Equipment

For strength development, intensity is the important variable, whereas for muscular endurance the duration of exercise assumes more importance.

In both strength training and aerobic conditioning it's often useful to use effort against resistance. This can range from resistance of the body against its own weight to complicated isokinetic machinery.

Some of this equipment is good, some not so good. In rating the equipment shown in Table 3.1, the following criteria were used to arrive at an evaluation of their usefulness:

- Effectiveness, i.e. for improving aerobic fitness, strength, power sport skills or muscle bulk; flexibility and body tension; reducing body fat.
- Safety.

- Ability to maintain motivation.
- Practicality and mechanical soundness.

Passive exercise machines: These include devices such as vibrating belts, vibrating pads, rollers, electric stimulators and sauna suits.

Because no effort is required by the exerciser, the only effect these machines have is (perhaps) relaxation. Research has shown, for example, that a person using a vibrating belt for 15 minutes every day for a year can expect to lose about 0.5 kg of body fat in that year — little more than would be lost standing still for the same amount of time.

According to the American Medical Association:

'The so called effortless exercisers have a value limited to the intensity and duration of the movement they demand. They do not provide any hidden benefits or values. Their most serious shortcoming is that most of them do very little to improve the fitness of the heart and lungs, which are most in need of exercise today.'

Weight training equipment: There are now many different forms of weight training equipment ranging from the traditional barbell/dumbells to elaborate machine systems. The latter all operate on slightly different biomechanical principles. All have their advantages and disadvantages and all can be excellent forms of conditioning if used properly.

Research shows that all systems are successful in the development of strength. The extent of improvement, however, depends on the measure of strength being used. If strength is assessed by variable resistance techniques, variable resistance training leads to approximately 20% greater improvement than constant resistance.

If assessment is through constant resistance techniques, the opposite is true. Improvements in body dimensions have also been shown to be roughly similar using fixed or variable resistance techniques. Hence the advantages claimed by various manufacturers do not always stand up to scrutiny.

Weights can be used for developing strength (heavy weights with low repetitions), for building body bulk (heavy to medium weights with 6–10 repetitions), or for developing cardiovascular fitness (light weights with high repetitions in circuit format).

Traditionally, because of the fear of developing muscle bulk, women have avoided resistance equipment. It is now accepted that large muscle development in women is generally limited by the lack of the male hormone testosterone, although it does occur in some cases.

Exercise bikes: In the gymnasium setting these are of the stationary type, but similar principles apply to moving bicycles.

Bikes can contribute an aerobic component to an exercise program. They can also be used for warming up and cooling down and for this reason alone are useful in an exercise area in a confined space.

Bikes can improve general fitness, leg strength and mobility in the knees and hips. They can reduce body fat and are especially useful for the obese or arthritic because they help support body weight.

Treadmills: An alternative to stationary cycling is stationary walking or jogging. Treadmill walking/running offers a good form of cardiovascular conditioning and can help burn up body fat. As with exercise bicycles, the main disadvantage of treadmills is the problem of maintaining motivation. They are useful for those who don't like running outdoors or during periods of poor weather and for the warm-up and cool-down phases of exercises in an indoor setting, but hold no other advantages over outdoor jogging.

Rowing machines: Rowing is an excellent form of aerobic exercise. It has an added advantage over running and cycling in that it uses the upper body and therefore increases the work effort and can contribute to upper body strength.

The problem of motivation noted above, however, is also true for rowing machines. For anyone but an experienced rower, the exercise can become boring over time — and this is not conducive to continued use.

Skipping ropes: Skipping is an exercise that's often highly regarded as a fitness tool. However, despite its long-term popularity, there have only been a limited number of scientific studies on its usefulness, and those that have been done question its overall effect. Research has pointed out that more energy is expended at a given exercise heart rate in jogging than skipping (at a heart rate of 70–80 bpm). This is because the energy requirement of an activity is largely dependent on the amount of muscle involved in that activity and jogging apparently uses more muscles than skipping in place.

In a more recent series of studies from Kent State University, blood lactate measures as well as oxygen uptake have been taken to test the involvement of different energy systems in skipping. The findings indicate that while five minutes of skipping at a rate of between 120–160 bpm can be quite strenuous, much of the energy used comes from anaerobic rather than aerobic sources. The resultant build-up of lactic acid in the blood stream means that the exercise can't be continued for long at that rate.

The implications are that it may be difficult to skip at a level which would give an effect equivalent to jogging for a period long enough to provide a training effect. In the gym situation it may be useful for warming up or as part of a circuit routine. It's unlikely, however, that it can be kept up long enough to be useful as a single conditioning technique.

Item	Claimed Benefits	Advantages	Disadvantages	Rating (out of 10)
Exercise bikes	Fitness/weight loss	Convenient, functional, useful for obese and arthritics	Can get boring, often poorly built	9
Treadmills	Fitness/weight loss	Indoor use in cold climates, functional, maximal exercise	Expense, can get boring, can cause joint soreness	8.5
Rowing machines	Fitness/weight loss/ strength	Good all round exercise, uses upper body, not space consuming	Can be boring and expensive	8
Weights	Strength/power/body bulk/fitness	Versatility, able to vary programs, wide range of equipment, fitness and strength component	Dangers if used incorrectly, space, expense	8.5
Mini-trampolines	Fitness	Novelty, less stress on weak joints of the lower limbs, not overly exerting for the less fit	Possible injury, motivation over a prolonged period	5.5
Skipping rope	Fitness/weight loss	Low cost, convenient	Boring, possible joint injuries	7
Saunas, steam baths, swirl pools	Weight loss/tension release	Relaxing	Do not lose weight, dangerous for some, i.e. with heart deficiencies, high blood pressure, may cause infections, allergies	1
Passive exercise equipment (rollers, pads, electric caps, sauna suits, etc.)	Weight loss	Minor massage effect	Some dangers, e.g. in pregnancy; no effect on weight or fitness, almost totally useless	0.5

Table 3.1: **Rating fitness equipment.**

Exercise Programming for Aerobic Conditioning

Although training and conditioning programs must be tailored to the individual, some basic principles apply for all people. In the first place, as we saw in Chapter 3, the most relevant type of exercises for the majority of the population are those defined by the S's: Stamina, Suppleness, Strength and Speed. In this chapter we'll concentrate on principles for developing stamina, or aerobic fitness. In Chapters 5 and 6 we'll look at suppleness, strength and speed development.

In recent years, there's been a vast amount of research aimed at clarifying issues concerning programming for physical activity. This can be summarised under the four headings with the acronym FITT (Frequency, Intensity, Time and Type), see Figure 4.1.

Frequency

In order to improve cardiovascular efficiency, a regular program of aerobic exercise should be carried out. Irregular mild exercise such as golf is ineffective in developing moderate levels of aerobic fitness.

Research has shown that above-average fitness can be maintained with regular workouts 3–4 times per week. Obviously more regular exercise will mean a higher level of fitness. However, for beginning exercisers this will have a training effect without causing significant discomfort, tiredness or boredom.

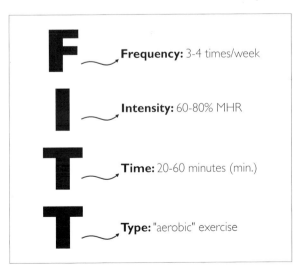

Figure 4.1: **Principles of exercise programming.**

During endurance training, total body mass and fat weight (FW) are reduced, while lean body mass (LBM) generally remains constant or increases slightly. Programs designed for fat loss should be carried out at a low to moderate intensity, 4–6 times per week for 20 to 60 minutes.

In order to maintain a training effect, exercise must be continued on a regular basis. There will be a significant reduction in fitness after two weeks of inactivity, with participants losing approximately 50% of their fitness after 4–12 weeks and 100% after 10–30 weeks.

Intensity

Because heart rate increases linearly with exercise effort, this is often used as a measure of the required intensity of exercise. Work carried out in Finland in the late 1950s showed that for noticeable gains in fitness, the heart rate during exercise should be raised by approximately 60% of the difference between the resting and maximal heart rates.

Other formulae set the training range at 70–85% of the age-estimated HR maximum. Figure 4.2 shows how this is determined. It has also been established that if improvements in general health and use of fat as fuel is the exercise goal, exercise intensity only needs to be moderate, ranging between 50% and 70% for the deconditioned and conditioned respectively.

Heart rate and exercise intensity

Heart rate can be monitored easily by periodically taking the pulse during an exercise session and then adjusting the exercise intensity to bring the heart rate to a recommended level. This recommended heart rate level is called the target heart rate. In most community-based exercise programs the two most common methods of determining desired exercise intensity are Karvonen's formula and the Perceived Rate of Exertion scale (PRE), shown on page 37.

The Karvonen Formula

The Karvonen Formula is a relatively accurate method of determining target heart rate. The formula calculates a percentage of the heart-rate reserve, which is the difference between the resting heart rate and maximal heart rate.

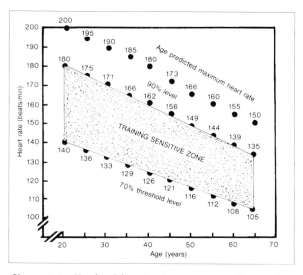

Figure 4.2: **Maximal heart rate target zone for use in aerobic exercise training (From Pyke, 1991)**

Maximal heart rate (MHR) is the highest heart rate a person can attain during heavy exercise. The most accurate way of determining maximal heart rate is to undergo a graded exercise test where the workload is continually increased until heart rate fails to increase in its normal linear fashion. In most instances this is not practical so the age-predicted maximum heart rate formula of 220 minus age is commonly used. Early research found that MHR peaked around the age of 20 years at about 200 bpm and declined approximately one beat per minute with each progressive year.

Demonstrated below is the use of Karvonen's Formula to calculate a heart rate range between 60% and 70% for a 42-year-old person with a resting heart rate of 85 bpm. The lower end of the target training range (60%) is 141 bpm or 23 bpm for a 10 second count and at 70% intensity is 150 bpm or 25 bpm for a 10 second count.

The steps for the Karvonen Formula are as follows:

1.	220 – 42 (age)	=	178 (MHR)
2.	178 (MHR) — 85 (RHR)	=	93 (HRR)
	a) 93 (HRR) x 0.60	=	55.8 + 85 (RHR) = 141 (THR)
	i) 141 (THR) / 6	=	23 beat 10 second heart rate
	b) 93 (HRR) x 0.70	=	65.1 + 85 (RHR) = 150 (THR)
	i) 150 (THR) / 6	=	25 beat 10 second heart rate

Abbreviations.

BPM = Beats per minute	RHR = Resting heart rate
HRR = Heart rate reserve	THR = Target heart rate
MHR = Maximum heart rate (220–age)	

The Karvonen Formula is a reasonably accurate way of determining target heart rate, with an error of + 5 to 10 beats per minute. It is recommended by the American College of Sports Medicine.

Perceived rate of exertion (PRE scale)

Intensity of effort can also be determined by using the Perceived Rate of Exertion Scale (see Table 4.1). This scale is especially relevant to those people who may have an unusually low or high heart rate, or those people who are on some form of medication that affects working heart rate. The PRE scale provides a means of quantifying subjective exercise intensity and have been found to correlate well (0.8 to 0.9) with oxygen uptake and heart rate. For the PRE scale to be used effectively perceptual anchors for the lower and upper levels should be established. For example, that a PRE of 0 is equivalent to quiet seated rest and that a PRE of 10 is equivalent to the most taxing physical effort the client can remember (Table 4.1).

The PRE chart should be placed in easy view of the exercising person, who should then be queried regularly as to the level of perceived exertion. Unless something out-of-the-ordinary comes up, exercise is considered to be maximal or near maximal when the exerciser reports a perceived exertion of 9 to 10.

0.	Nothing at all	5.	Strong
0.5	Very, very weak	6.	
1.	Very weak	7.	Very strong
2.	Weak	8.	
3.	Moderate	9.	
4.	Somewhat strong	10.	Very, very strong — Maximal

Table 4.1: **Perceived rate of exertion (PRE) chart.**

The talk test

Another simple test of intensity to ensure that the heart rate reaches a count of 120–130 bpm during exercise is the talk test. This sets a safe lower value for the establishment of a training effect at most ages. At the higher level, the 'talk test' can be used to assess whether an individual is working out too hard. If the exerciser can't comfortably talk (or whistle) while exercising, the effort is more than likely anaerobic and therefore of greater intensity than

necessary for an aerobic training effect. For beginning exercisers it is unwise to continue at this level.

Pulse-taking techniques

The most common errors that occur in recording intensity using heart rate include miscounting and taking too long to begin counting. Therefore, fitness instructors should be familiar with all the procedures for taking heart rates.

The two most common places for palpating and recording heart rate are the wrist and the neck.

Wrist: The radial pulse can be felt on the radial artery of the wrist, in line with the thumb. Place the tips of the index and middle fingers (not the thumb, which has a pulse of its own) and press down slightly.

Neck: The carotid pulse can be felt on the carotid artery, which is located on the neck just to the side of the trachea. Place the first two fingers gently on the side of the neck. Too much pressure placed on the carotid artery may stimulate a reflex mechanism that causes the heart to slow down.

The pulse can be taken for 6 seconds (and multiplied by 10), for 10 seconds (and multiplied by 6), or for 15 seconds (and multiplied by 4).

It is recommended that the first pulse be counted as 1 and the pulse be taken for 10 seconds. Because heart rate begins to decrease soon after exercise stops, instructors should begin the count as soon as possible, preferably within 5 seconds.

Time

The minimum length of time of an exercise session for significant improvements in aerobic fitness is 20–60 minutes. Improved performance will continue (within reason) the longer the exercise session is continued. Beyond an hour, the returns start to become less. It is at this level that one might train if competition is the desired end.

For a beginning exerciser, it's often unwise to continue an exercise session beyond 30 minutes at an intensity greater than 60%. Sessions should be limited to 15–20 minutes. If necessary, recovery periods of 1–2 minutes can be included between the heavier segments of activity.

Exercise	Weight control	Sleep	Digestion	Cardiovascular endurance	Approx. energy use per minute (calories)
Walking	8	6	5	6	5-7
Jogging	10*	8*	6	10*	12-16
Swimming	5	8*	7*	10*	6-11
Cycling	9	8*	6	10*	8-15
Tennis	6	5	6	7	5-11
Golf (walking)	3	3	5	4	5-8
Skiing (downhill)	5	8*	6	6	6-10
Stepping/Skipping/Jumping	7	5	5	7	5-11
Surfing	6	8*	7*	10*	6-11
Step Classes	8	7	7*	9	9-14
Aerobic Classes	8	7	7	9	9-14
Handball/Squash	8	6	7*	10*	10-15
Canoeing	7	8*	6	8	4-10

* Signifies the best exercise(s) for that purpose. Energy use increases with body weight. These figures are based on an approximate body weight of 70 kg.

Table 4.2: **Rating (out of 10) for a variety of exercise effects.**

Type

The type of aerobic activities that develop cardiovascular endurance are those that involve the use of 50% or more of the body's muscle mass and can be carried out continuously at a sustained rate (e.g. aerobically). The relative values of various activities depend on the amount of effort required (see Table 4.2). For example, golf, bowls, archery and doubles tennis may be recreational and enjoyable, but they do little for aerobic fitness. Vigorous, continuous and rhythmic activities on the other hand, like swimming, jogging, cross country skiing, cycling, canoeing, dancing and brisk walking are all potentially aerobic if carried out to the FITT formula.

A wide variety of aerobic activities can be carried out either individually or in groups. For example:

On your own

These are the simplest forms of activity because they don't require dependence on another person. They generally call for little elaborate equipment or expense, and can help an individual feel in control of his/her own programming.

Activities include: walking, jogging, cycling, swimming, skating, weight training, skipping, golf, rowing.

Comparisons of some of these (e.g. running and swimming) as training techniques have shown that where equivalent intensities are used (i.e. equal exercise heart rates), both are equally efficient in developing cardiovascular fitness, although it has been estimated that the distance ratio between running and swimming is roughly 5:1, i.e. a 5 km run equals a 1 km swim.

Instructor-based

Many aerobic activities provide the stimulation of a group working out under the direction of an inspired leader. These may be indoor or outdoor, and with or without the added benefit of music. Classes are most suitable for those who prefer social interaction, who find it tedious organising their own routines, and who respond best to the motivating influences of others.

Activities include:, aerobic classes, step classes, aquarobics, modern dance, and circuit classes.

Studies of aerobics classes have shown that the effort required over 60 minutes of dancing is equivalent to an extended bout of jogging or cycling. Where heart rates are elevated to 120–140 bpm, the energy required is roughly equivalent to running at around a 10-minute-mile pace. Aerobic class dancing is twice as strenuous as more traditional dancing, but perhaps less so than aerobic exercise to music.

One-on-one

For some people, competition provides the motivation for aerobic activity. Competitive games are often a source of fun and enjoyment that can help to develop reflexes and specific skills as well as general aerobic fitness. The key to adequate aerobic exercise through competitive games is for both competitors to be similar in standard. This ensures that players are then kept continuously active.

Activities include: tennis, squash, badminton, racquetball, table tennis, boxing.

Evaluation of the energy components of various racquet sports shows that these are of varying value in improving aerobic fitness. Singles tennis, for example, may be a reasonable way for a beginner to improve initial fitness levels, but will not sufficiently overload someone of advanced fitness. Squash, handball and badminton, conversely, are beneficial for skilled players who can keep the ball in play, but less so for beginners.

Team games

Team sports combine the benefits of class activities and competitive games. Like class activities, they turn fitness into a social event, and the competitive element can be extremely stimulating.

Activities include: basketball, volleyball, soccer, football, touch football, hockey, cricket, netball, water polo, softball, surf lifesaving.

In many of these (e.g. volleyball, cricket, softball) the action is stop-go, hence significant anaerobic or phosphate components are involved; thus these games, while providing social stimulation, are not good fitness builders. Best for aerobic conditioning are those games that require constant movement throughout the game, e.g. soccer, hockey, basketball, water polo.

Getting away

Certain outdoor activities combine adventure, fresh air and open skies with fitness-enhancing activity. These can vary according to season, location and availability of time. However, to be effective aerobic conditioners they should be carried out regularly (i.e. a minimum of three times a week) or combined with other events.

Activities include skiing, surfing, mountain climbing, bush walking, orienteering, canoeing, rowing, and windsurfing.

Research has shown that cross-country skiing is perhaps the best form of aerobic conditioning available. It rates even higher than jogging because of the use of the large muscles of the arms as well as the legs. Downhill skiing rates less highly because of its stop-start nature and the short intense periods involved.

For an individual to continue an exercise program over a lifetime, that program has to be enjoyable. Hence, selection of the appropriate exercise is important. This can be done from a detailed interview or through completion of a questionnaire such as that shown in Figure 4.3.

Variety can also be important for motivation. A combination of aerobic activities carried out to the FITT plan will be as effective in developing cardiovascular conditioning as the continuation of one type of exercise only. For example, a typical fortnightly routine may follow that outlined in Table 4.3.

In winter, an activity like cycling could substitute for swimming.

An added advantage to this type of program for a beginning exerciser is that it provides the opportunity for the exerciser to later select and concentrate on the preferred types of exercise.

Exercise Prescription

Any exercise program must be designed and evaluated on an individual basis. Anyone designing such a program should consider the following:

Age: The period of maximum maturity is between 25 and 30, with an acceleration in decline after age 50. As a person ages, improvement and recovery are slower, as are de-conditioning and re-conditioning. Prescription of exercise for the aged therefore must take into consideration the previous level of activity of the individual as well as any specific musculoskeletal problems that may limit the type of exercises possible.

Day	Week 1	Week 2
Monday	Jogging	Jogging
Tuesday	Swimming	Circuit training
Wednesday	Circuit training	Swimming
Thursday	Jogging	Jogging
Friday	Swimming	Circuit training
Saturday	Circuit training	Swimming
Sunday	Rest	Rest

Table 4.3: **A typical 2-week regime.**

Gender: There are general absolute strength differences between men and women. Women have approximately two-thirds the general muscular strength of men. This difference between genders is mainly attributed to the positive relationship of strength to muscle size. However, when compared for ability to exert force per unit of muscle mass, there is little or no difference between sexes, and this also applies to muscular endurance.

Gains in muscular strength are usually accompanied by an increase in the size of muscle fibres. While this is true for both sexes, it is much less pronounced in females. Because of the absence of the male hormone testosterone, most women won't experience significant muscle bulking (hypertrophy) in response to resistance exercise.

In terms of cardiovascular function, women have a higher heart rate (5–10 bpm faster) than men, and it has been shown that women have 80–90% of the aerobic capacity of men. However, when body composition is taken into consideration and measurement is based on the same amount of active muscle this difference diminishes significantly.

Generally speaking, women are more flexible than men. Hence some stretching-type exercises, while suitable for the females, can put extra strain on males. The competitive nature of many men also makes for added danger if the man doesn't accept his limitations.

INSTRUCTIONS FOR EXERCISE SELECTOR QUESTIONNAIRE

1. Circle the number under each exercise corresponding to the answer in each category. Add scores down the column for each exercise to get your total test scores.

2. Calculate your Interest Score for each activity. If you think you'd enjoy carrying out the activity regularly, give yourself an Interest Score of 100. If you think you may enjoy carrying out the activity regularly, give yourself an Interest Score of 90. If the activity doesn't appeal, give yourself an Interest Score of 80.

3. Calculate a final score for each activity by subtracting the Total Test Score from the Interest Score for each activity.

4. The activity with the highest final score will generally be the most appropriate aerobic exercise for you. If there are several activities at the top falling within about 5 points of each other, choose the one you think you would prefer. Or combine them as part of the one program.

Personal Details	Jogging	Cycling	Swimming	Dancing	Skipping	Ball Games
Age:						
Under 35	0	0	0	0	0	0
35–49	0	0	0	1	3	4
50–59	2	3	0	3	5	5
60+	4	7	0	4	8	6
Body Frame:						
Small/medium	0	0	0	0	0	0
Large	3	0	0	2	4	2
Are you … more than a little overweight?						
No	0	0	0	0	0	0
Yes	4	3	0	4	5	6
… an indoor or outdoor type person?						
Indoor	7	6	4	0	0	4
Outdoor	0	1	2	0	5	0
… self-conscious about exercising in public?						
No	0	0	0	0	0	0
Yes	5	4	4	7	0	5
… competitive?						
Very	3	5	3	8	8	0
Moderately	0	4	3	5	5	2
Not very	0	2	3	0	0	8
… prepared to pay more than $10 a week to exercise?						
Yes	0	0	0	0	0	0
No	0	2	1	4	0	4
… suffering limiting injuries to any of the following?						
Legs/ankles/knees	9	4	1	7	9	7
shoulders/arms	1	2	3	2	4	5
hip	9	3	3	7	8	7
back	5	5	2	6	5	6
… not within easy access (say 15 mins) of any of the following?						
pool/lake/sea	0	0	10	0	0	0
park/open space	5	0	0	0	0	0
gymnasium	0	0	0	3	0	4
sports facilities	0	0	0	0	0	10
safe bike routes	0	10	0	0	0	0
… prepared to give up daily time 3–4 days a week?						
less than 20 mins	4	5	10	10	3	10
20–40 mins	0	1	4	2	0	4
more than 40 mins	0	0	0	0	0	0
… a person who prefers … ?						
exercising alone	0	0	0	5	0	10
with a friend	1	2	2	0	3	0
in a group	2	4	2	0	6	0
Total Test Score:						
Interest Score:						
FINAL SCORE:						

Figure 4.3: **Exercise Selector Questionnaire: Selecting the form of exercise most appropriate for an individual.**

SAMPLE LIFESTYLE SCREENING QUESTIONNAIRE

Name:	Age:	Sex:
Address:	P/Code:	
Occupation:	Phone H:	Phone W:

Please complete only Parts A and B of this questionnaire.

Part A: Your goals and current exercise habits.

1. Please ✔ what you hope to achieve from your exercise program:
   - To reduce body fat ❑
   - To improve aerobic capacity (heart/lung fitness) ❑
   - To gain some muscle definition ❑
   - To gain overall fitness ❑
   - To generally tone up ❑
   - To reduce stress ❑
   - Other_____

2. In order for us to help you achieve your goals, please ✔ if you would like us to:
   - Provide you with personalised service? Yes ❑ No ❑
   - Contact you if you miss training sessions? Yes ❑ No ❑
   - Leave you alone so you can train when it suits you? Yes ❑ No ❑

3. To help us tailor an excercise program to your specific needs, please answer the following questions concerning your exercise history.
   - While at school did you enjoy participating in sporting programs? Yes ❑ No ❑
   - If yes, which sports were your favourites?
   - Have you been exercising regularly? Yes ❑ No ❑ __mths___Yrs
   - If you have been exercising regularly please give details below:
     (1) Type of exercise:
     (II) Frequency of exercise — times per week:
     (III) Perceived intensity when exercising:
     Hard ❑
     Medium ❑
     Light ❑
     Very Light ❑
   - Do you have any negative feelings or have you had any bad experiences with exercise programs? Yes ❑ No ❑
     If yes, please briefly explain:

Part B: Lifestyle and medical considerations. Please answer with a ✔ the following questions:
   - Are you taking any prescribed medication? Yes ❑ No ❑
   - Are you currently carrying an injury? Yes ❑ No ❑
   - Have you suffered or do suffer from back pain? Yes ❑ No ❑
   - Do you smoke more than 2 cigarettes a day? Yes ❑ No ❑
   - Are you pregnant? Yes ❑ No ❑
   - Are you a non-exercising male over 35 or female over 45? Yes ❑ No ❑
   - Do you know your blood pressure? Yes ❑ No ❑
     If yes, what is it? ___/___
   - Do you suffer from asthma attacks? Yes ❑ No ❑
   - Do you suffer from diabetes? Yes ❑ No ❑
   - Has anyone in your family under the age of 60 suffered heart disease? Yes ❑ No ❑

Part C: Heath Screening (Do not complete this section unless asked to by your trainer).
Please indicate with a ✔ whether you have or have had any of the following:

Gout	❑	Glandular fever	❑	Any heart condition	❑
Stroke	❑	Rheumatic fever	❑	Heart murmur	❑
Asthma	❑	Dizziness or fainting	❑	High blood pressure more than 140/90	❑
Epilepsy	❑	Stomach or duodenal ulcer	❑	Chest pain	❑
Hernia	❑	Liver or kidney problems	❑	Raised cholesterol	❑

Trainer's comments:

I understand that an exercise program has certain risks. I take it upon myself to discuss any changes in my current health with the staff.
I have to the best of my knowledge provided accurate information regarding my current health status.

Signed   Date

Figure 4.4: **A suggested questionnaire to be completed before exercise prescription.**

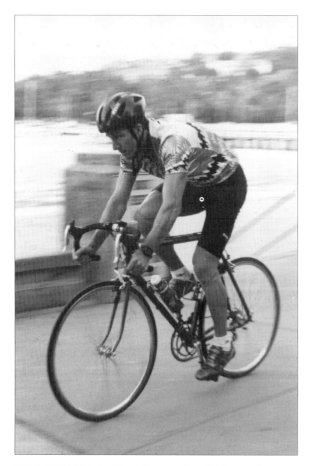

For a person to continue to exercise, that exercise must be enjoyable. Cycling is increasing in popularity as an efficient and satisfying way to burn energy.

Previous activity and conditioning experience: Although there are no residual benefits to exercise once a program has been discontinued, the individual who has had previous training experience is likely to respond more quickly to training than one who has not. That person will also usually achieve a higher level of fitness or skill.

Psychological factors and motivation: Each individual enters a training program with pre-determined perceptions regarding exercise, his or her level of skill, ability to learn and ability to endure a particular training regimen. Often the amount of improvement is limited more by psychological factors than by actual physical capacity. An instructor must therefore recognise and address this through motivational and human relations skills. Conversely, an individual's drive may exceed his or her physical capacities, and this may have to be curbed.

Fitness assessment: Objective fitness assessment is a key ingredient in any successful exercise program. A series of assessment tests that can be used in the practical situation is outlined in Chapter 10.

Individual needs: Fitness evaluation procedures will establish specifically the areas of emphasis that need to be addressed in designing an exercise program. These include such things as time available, specific interests and health problems.

These factors should all be assessed before prescribing an exercise program. The screening questionnaire shown in Figure 4.4 is one way of doing this as a prelude to the more detailed assessment tests of Chapter 10.

Health and lifestyle screening: An instructor can obtain a considerable amount of information about a client from a comprehensive lifestyle and pre-exercise screening questionnaire (see Fig. 4.4 and Chapter 10).

In addition, such screening questionnaires will: (1) help identify medical conditions that may place the client at risk; (2) highlight the client's exercise objectives; (3) identify whether there are any activities that are unsuitable to the client; (4) assist in the development of an exercise program that will fulfill the client's needs.

Health Status: This will obviously determine the amount and intensity of overload and the rate of progression of an exercise program. Overload and intensity should be reduced even during minor illnesses such as a cold or minor infection. Since the body under such conditions is already under stress, further physical stress should be avoided.

Present level of condition: This will determine the starting point of an exercise program, and be reflected in the rate of improvement. The less fit a person is, the greater the improvement that can be shown. Conversely, the closer a person is to his or her maximum performance, the less improvement will be shown, and more effort will be required to make noticeable gains.

Planning a Workout

Once all of the above factors are considered, emphasis needs to be given to the way in which an aerobic program can be tailored to a client's needs. All programs should consist of three essential parts: 1. the warm-up phase 2. the conditioning phase 3. the cool-down phase. Together these make up the Three-segment Workout.

The warm-up

A gentle warm-up should always precede strenuous activity. The purpose of this is:

* To stimulate the heart and lungs moderately and progressively.
* To increase blood flow.
* To increase body temperature gradually and increase the metabolism of skeletal muscle.
* To help prevent muscle and joint injury.
* To prepare psychologically for the effort to follow.

An effective warm-up consists of two parts:

1. General warm-up: This involves rhythmic movement of the entire body in order to increase circulation and body temperature. The time required will vary with the individual and the outside temperature. However, the commencement of sweating indicates that the body is ready for more vigorous activity.

2. Specific warm-up: This involves stretches and movements that will be specifically used in the activities to follow. Specific warm-up should aid in the prevention of muscle strain. The actual skill to be used later should be performed at medium speed. Numerous examples of specific warm-up can be seen prior to sporting events. Some warm-up stretches for various sports are shown in Figure 4.5. Other stretches are shown in Chapter 5.

The conditioning bout

The recommended activities for cardiovascular conditioning and weight control are those aerobic exercises listed in Table 4.2. These stimulate the cardiovascular system to induce a training effect. All exercise should be conducted according to the FITT principle.

The cool-down

This is the tapering-off period. It is important to maintain the muscles' ability to return blood from the extremities to the heart. Following an exercise session a large supply of blood remains in the working muscles. If this is not returned promptly to the central circulation, pooling of the blood may occur in the muscles. If the brain doesn't receive sufficient blood fainting can occur.

Cooling down is best accomplished by a continuation of the activity at a lower intensity. Generally this involves keeping moving by walking or light jogging for some five minutes after exercise. Gentle movement should continue until the heart rate returns to a steady state. Static and PNF stretching should be included at the end of the cool-down. In fact, recent research suggests that greatest flexibility gains are achieved as a result of flexibility training following the exercise session.

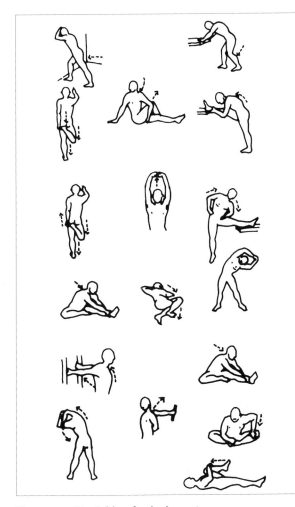

Figure 4.5: **Stretching for body parts.**

Planning a Circuit Program

Circuit training is the arrangement of known and proven exercises designed to elicit maximum overall training effectiveness. Circuit training has as its objective the development of strength, endurance and cardiorespiratory fitness. It aims at overall fitness rather than specific fitness for different activities.

Over the past few years circuit training has gained enormous popularity in fitness centres. The following could account for this:

* It adds variety to an individual's training program.
* It does not discriminate between men and women.
* It is a good introduction for people wishing to commence a weight training program.
* It makes very efficient use of equipment.
* It accommodates different fitness levels.
* It adds a specific muscular endurance component to the training session.
* It incorporates all of the four S's of fitness.

There are two ways of planning a circuit:

Method 1: This involves using fixed resistance, fixed repetitions and minimising the time taken to complete the circuit. 'Parcourse' programs in parks are examples of this method. The main advantage is that it is easy to monitor improvement by recording the time taken to complete the circuit.

Method 2: In this case each exercise is carried out with a fixed resistance for as many repetitions as possible in a given period of time. The circuit class is an example of this method. The main advantage is that participants can work at their own pace without having to wait before stations. The use of the circuit timer will facilitate this method.

Exercise layout

The exercises in any circuit should be laid out in specific order to enhance the training effect and prevent overload of specific muscle groups. This can be done by:

* alternating exercises to different body parts. For example, a leg press can be followed by an arm curl; sit-ups followed by a leg curl;
* using a large-muscle activity between exercises,

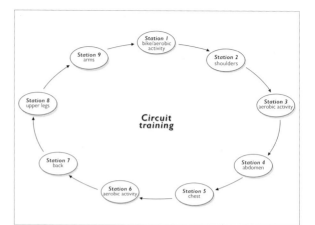

Figure 4.6: **Arrangement of a nine-station circuit.**

which will increase the aerobic effect of the circuit. For example, running, cycling, mini-trampolining or step-ups.

Circuit training can be extremely demanding and beginners can very easily develop feelings of nausea and discomfort. As a result it is advisable that all beginners are:

* adequately screened (see Fig. 4.4);
* taught the correct exercise technique;
* taught how to monitor perceived rate of exertion effectively;
* warned against over-competitiveness;
* informed of the importance of warming up and cooling down.

Participant benefits

The benefits of circuit training for the participant are:

* It provides a compromise between aerobic and strength training.
* It avoids overuse problems such as repetitive foot strike patterns.
* It provides a balanced program of strength development.
* It is not intimidating for people who have not used weights previously.
* It is a time-effecient workout.
* It encourages group involvment.
* It can be easily adapted to suit different age groups and fitness levels.
* It is an overall energy burner.
* It can be adapted to meet the specific needs of different sports.

- It is an effective fitness program for people recovering from injury.
- Its structure can be regularly changed to maintain participant motivation.

Fitness centre benefits

The benefits of incorporating circuit training into the exercise options provided by a fitness centre are:

- It suites a large cross section of the exercising public.
- It is very space-efficient.
- It is easier to instruct than an aerobic class.
- It provides a vehicle through which hardened resistance trainers can do some aerobic work in a non-threatening environment. This also applies to aerobic enthusiasts who wish to do some weight training.
- It is less physically demanding on the instructor, thereby reducing instructor burnout.
- It promotes a very positive gym atmosphere.

Circuit Variables

When designing a circuit there are three important variables that can be manipulated to alter the training emphasis of the program — the resistance, the set duration, and the rest duration.

Resistance: The amount of resistance will depend upon the equipment used, the desired training effect and the strength of participants.

Set Duration: The time allowed to perform each exercise can vary between 20 and 60 seconds, to suit the fitness levels of participants and training objectives of the circuit.

Rest Duration: The recovery period between exercises can be increased or decreased to meet the desired training intensity. For example:

General conditioning	0–10 secs.
Strength and power	30–60 secs.
Older or very unfit	20–60 secs.

Other variables that can be manipulated in a circuit program are the duration of the circuit and the intensity at which each exercise is completed.

Following are two different types of circuit that are inexpensive and require little space. The first requires a few free weights and a timer. The second is even more basic and needs only a few sheets of paper, pencil and a bank of exercises.

Circuits using free weights, machines and equipment

To ensure the circuit has an adequate aerobic component, exercises should be carried out with light weights and high repetitions (15–20), and preferably include the larger muscle groups.

Free weight circuit: Examples of exercises for a free weight circuit incorporating some equipment are:

- Squat
- Bicep curl
- Exercise bike
- Bench press
- Abdominal crunch
- Power clean
- Mini trampoline
- Upright row
- Abdominal crunch
- Press behind neck
- Exercise bike
- Pullovers
- Lunges
- Dumbbell flyes
- Skipping

Machine system equipment circuit: These circuits are becoming more popular, with fitness centres establishing specific circuit rooms using a range of equipment. The machines systems used for circuits can be divided into two broad categories, those using hydraulic cylinders and those using cams and cables.

Non-equipment circuits: This type of circuit is a good substitute for an aerobic class as most participants will be familiar with the exercises. Examples of exercise stations that can be used are:

- Squats with lateral raise
- Push-ups with hands wide
- Tuck jumps
- Abdominal crunch

- Forward lunge (alternate legs)
- Side leg lifts (left side)
- Push-ups with hands close
- Reverse curl
- Side leg lifts (right side)
- Dips
- Free squats
- Karate punches
- Reverse lunge (alternate legs)
- Step ups

All the above exercises can be interspersed with aerobic movements such as running on the spot, skipping, travelling moves, push backs, etc.

1. Prime mover circuit:

In this format circuit participants work in pairs. For example, on station 1, participant A completes a set of supine flye exercises while participant B, on station 2, completes a set of bench presses. At the end of the set period (i.e. 40 secs) the participants then swap exercises. This can then be repeated a second or even third time.

Station 1	Station 2
Supine Flys Dumbbell	Bentover Row
Bench Press Barbell	Dumbbell Row
Station 3	**Station 4**
Step-ups Dumbbell	Upright Row Barbell
Squats Dumbbell or Barbell	Shrugs Dumbbell
Station 5	**Station 6**
Tricep Extension Dumbbell	Lunges Dumbbell
Tricep Extension Barbell	Deadlifts Barbell
Station 7	**Station 8**
Bicep Curls Dumbbell	Front Raise Dumbbell
Bicep Curls Barbell	Side Raises Dumbbell
Station 9	**Station 10**
Calves Barbell	Back Extensions Barbell
Calves Dumbbell	Back Extensions
Station 11	**Station 12**
Crunches	Wrist Flexion
Pelvic tilts	Wrist Extension

2. Agonist/antagonist circuit:

The same procedure is followed as for the prime mover circuit; however, in this circuit the exercises are arranged so that the agonist muscle is being followed by the antagonist muscle.

Station 1	Station 2
Bench press	Squats
Bentover Row	Deadlifts
Station 3	**Station 4**
Bicep Curl	Front Raises
Tricep Extension	Dumbell Row (elbow in)
Station 5	**Station 6**
Upright Row	Crunches
Pullovers	Extensions

3. Recovery circuit:

Same procedures as for the the above two circuits but here the exercises are organised so that different body parts are being worked. This allows for sufficient recovery time between stations.

Station 1	Station 2
Squats	Biceps Curl
Bentover Row	Bench Press
Station 3	**Station 4**
Crunches	Lunges
Shoulder Press	Pullovers
Station 5	**Station 6**
Tricep Extensions	Calf Raises
Back Extensions	Shrugs

Participant motivation

Circuit classes like aerobic classes must provide variety to ensure that participants stay motivated. Some techniques that the instructor can use are:

Music selection: If used the selected music should have an energetic sound and can vary from 140–170 bpm. Generally speaking the music should be selected from more traditional tracks, while having a stronger sound than would normally be heard on an aerobic floor. The warm-up music should have a range of 130–137 bpm.

Varying the exercise sequence: There are a number of ways an instructor can change the sequence of exercises to provide variety. Examples are: changing the direction of the circuit, skipping a station, doubling up on a station and moving from the normal circuit format into lines for floor work.

Include a competitive aspect: This is suited to more experienced participants. The instructor sets a target number of repetitions per station that the participants attempt to attain.

General considerations for all circuits

Space: Most circuits can be adapted to the allocated space. However, instructors should ensure that there is sufficient space between participants.

Music: The music selected must be motivational and should vary depending on the type of circuit.

Beginners: If possible, give beginners some instruction on exercise technique before the circuit commences. Also, it is a good idea to place a beginner next to an experienced participant so that he/she can see how the exercise should be performed.

Length of time at each station: The ideal time per station is 30 seconds. However, it is important to encourage participants to move from one station to another as quickly as possible to get the greatest benefit from the allocated time.

Heart rate checks: As a general rule take a heart rate check after 15 minutes, at the end of the circuit, and after the cool-down.

Checkpoint

Fitness instructors should take into consideration the following when designing and leading a circuit using floor class exercises:

- Do the participants know how to correctly execute each exercise?
- Does the circuit meet the right safety guidelines?
- Is the circuit well balanced to ensure all the major muscles are overloaded?
- Is there too much repetitive foot strike in the aerobic movements?
- Have the selected exercises been properly sequenced?

Fitness instructors should take into consideration the following when leading a machine circuit:

- Does all the equipment work properly?
- What level of resistance is the equipment set at? Does the equipment need to be wiped down after each person?
- Do all the participants know how to use each piece of apparatus?
- Do any of the participants have any limitations with regard to use of any of the equipment?

Guidelines for Aerobic Exercise Programs

The following are suggested standards for conducting aerobic exercise programs:

* The session must have a genuine aerobic component that lasts for a minimum of 20 minutes at an intensity measured preferably for a minimum heart rate of 120 bpm.
* Participants should be encouraged to carry out such an exercise at least 3 times per week.
* At least 5 minutes must be spent performing a range of motion stretching and warming up at the start of the program, and slow static stretching and cooling down at the end.
* Progression from warm-up to aerobic effort must be gradual, as it should also be with cool-down.
* Ballistic (bouncy) movements should be avoided as much as possible during the progression of the program, particularly for inexperienced exercisers.
* As far as possible, classes should be structured to cater for beginner and advanced exercisers, with separate classes conducted for each.
* All new participants in a class should be questioned as to their previous exercise levels and advised as to the level recommended for their purpose.
* Attention must be given to the correct procedures in carrying out specific exercises.
* Advice should be given to certain clients about the level of difficulty of some exercises (many men have difficulty with certain flexibility exercises more suited to women – adductor/abductor stretches, back flexes, etc.).
* Advice should be given on the type of clothing to wear to prevent over-heating or chafing.
* If classes are carried out to music, this should be such as to ensure a slow and gradual warm-up of at least 5 minutes and a similar cool-down.
* Precautions must be taken at all times to prevent both acute and chronic injury. This includes the overuse of certain techniques such as bouncing on toes, or running with bare feet on hard surfaces.
* Participants should be advised from the start of the program as to how long the exercise period will be and of any idiosyncrasies in the program that may not be expected.
* Participants must be asked if they are taking any form of medication, and if so, what this may be. Where no knowledge about a medication is immediately available, steps should be taken to ascertain contraindications, if any.
* Participants should be advised to exercise before rather than after eating; but limited non-alcoholic fluid intake before, and even during, prolonged exercise is advisable.
* Special attention should be paid to the possibility of dehydration in hot weather (see Chapter 2).
* All participants should be encouraged to wear well cushioned shoes in activities involving running, skipping or hopping.
* Participants must never be allowed to join classes when they have not had sufficient warm-up.

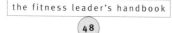

Exercise Programming for Suppleness and Flexibility Training

Suppleness (flexibility) refers to the range of motion or movement of a joint or group of joints. Although this may be affected by structural damage to the bones of the joint, the most common factor affecting flexibility is the inability of the muscles surrounding a joint to stretch to an optimal length.

In most people, joints have the potential to move through a greater range of motion than the muscles that surround them will allow. Through regular stretching the muscles' capacity to extend fully is increased, thus allowing the joint a greater range of motion.

Flexibility is an important factor in all aspects of human movement, particularly sports-related activities. Limited flexibility results in restricted movement and a greater possibility of injury; many studies and observations show that the more flexible athletes are better performers in their sport.

Flexibility is improved by reduced muscle tension, using controlled force to increase the range of movement, and lengthening the connective tissue.

Why Stretch?

Without regular stretching, muscles tend to lose flexibility so that when called upon to perform an extreme movement, as in an emergency, they are less able to extend to their full range of movement, often resulting in damage to the muscle tissue.

Proper stretching, even for short periods, can help in the following ways:

Prevent injuries: Stretching improves the range of movement of a muscle. Hence, if a joint is stretched to its limit, a muscle with a greater capacity to lengthen will allow greater movement.

Improve biomechanical efficiency: An example is a tight achilles tendon. It is inefficient because it does not allow a complete and strong push-off for each stride during running.

Increase extensibility of muscles: Increasing

range of movement allows for greater speed and power in actions that require a wide range, e.g. throwing in baseball, bowling in cricket.

Improve co-ordination between muscle groups: Where variability exists in opposing muscle groups weaknesses can develop in musculo-tendinous connections.

Improve relaxation of muscles: This is often an advantage for pre-competition warm-up, helping the athlete feel psychologically prepared for the action to follow.

Decrease muscle tightening after movement: Stretching after the event can diminish muscle tightening and prevent stiffness (not soreness) developing.

Counteract the possible restricting effects of hypertrophy training: For some sports, muscle bulking is desirable, but this can have the effect of shortening muscles that aren't put through their full range of movement. Stretching helps alleviate the problem.

Factors Affecting Flexibility

A variety of factors can affect flexibility. These include:

Exercise: Active people tend to be more flexible.

Heat: An increase in temperature induced by either direct heat or the weather can increase the range of motion and elasticity of a muscle. Conversely, a decrease in temperature can result in a decrease in flexibility of as much as 20%. This illustrates the need for adequate warm-up and stretching before activities such as ice skating, skiing and swimming.

Age: Stiffness is often associated with advancing age. Muscle contractability remains, while elasticity is lost, resulting in tighter, stiffer muscles. A reduction in activity also decreases flexibility. Hence, increasing activity and muscle stretching can keep the effects of these changes to a minimum.

Warming up: Warming up produces an increase in muscle temperature. The flexibility of joints and muscles is more easily achieved after an adequate warm-up period.

Gender: Most comparative studies have shown females to be more flexible than males in most joints, and remain so throughout adult life. It is not known quite why this is so, but it has been attributed to the different training experiences of boys and girls early in life.

Specificity: Flexibility is specific to each joint and the angle of contraction of the muscles surrounding (or supporting) the joint. Hence flexibility programs should concentrate on those areas of the body that are to be involved in specific activity, though the 'unused' muscles should not be neglected.

Types of Stretching

Stretching exercises fall into four broad categories:

1. Passive stretching is sometimes referred to as static stretching. This form of stretching involves the gradual stretching of a muscle to a point where it is held, without bouncing, for 15 to 30 seconds. The muscle should be taken to a point where there is a feeling in the muscle that it is being stretched. If the muscle is taken to the point of discomfort then the tension should be eased off.

Static stretching is a safe and effective way of stretching muscles and connective tissue. Because it involves no sudden movements it does not provoke the stretch reflex as much as in ballistic stretching.

Static stretching is best suited for:
- general stretching of all muscles;
- the early stages of recovery from injury;
- the cool-down phase following a vigorous exercise program.

2. Range of motion stretching: (ROM) sometimes referred to as dynamic or active stretching. This form of stretching arose out of the concern that some people tend to overstretch in a passive or PNF (see category 4) situation. This may cause damage to the muscle and tendon fibres, particularly in the case of recovery from over-use injuries, such as tendonitis.

ROM stretching has become an integral part of the warm-up of most aerobic classes. It involves the rhythmical movement of the major muscles that will be used in the exercise program. ROM stretches should be gentle repetitions of the types of movements that will be experienced in the workout.

Active stretching is best suited for:

🏃 stretching immediately before a period of vigorous activity (such as an exercise class to music);

🏃 stretching the muscle groups that cross the major joints (such as the shoulders, the hips, the knees and ankles).

3. Ballistic stretching:
This form of stretching is bounce stretching, where the muscle is taken to the end of its range of motion, and then over-stretched by bouncing. In the past this was a common way of stretching, but has now been discarded because of a knowledge of the intra-muscular damage that may occur as a result of the 'stretch reflex'.

The stretch reflex:
Muscle fibres contain sensory nerve endings called muscle spindles (see Chapter 2) whose main function is to send messages back from the muscle to inform the central nervous system about its state of stretch.

If the muscle is stretched abruptly, distortion of the central part of the muscle spindle causes the stretch reflex to automatically come into play, causing the muscle to contract, thus avoiding damage through tearing.

The amount and rate of contraction elicited from the stretch reflex are proportional to the amount and rate of stretching. Hence, the faster and more forceful the stretch, the faster and more forceful the reflex contraction of the stretched muscle, and thus the likelihood of the muscle tearing — particularly in an untrained muscle. For this reason bouncing, or 'ballistic', actions in exercise programs are not recommended. However, ballistic exercises may be important in the well-conditioned athlete who may require ballistic and explosive actions in his/her sport. But in this case, actions should be preceded by either passive or ROM stretching.

4. PNF stretching:
PNF stands for Proprioceptive Neuromuscular Facilitation. Although relatively recent in fitness training, PNF has been used in the rehabilitation of muscle and tendon injury for some time. A variation of this has now become the most accepted form of stretching for best results in flexibility training and injury prevention.

Research has shown that back flexion as measured by a sit-and-reach test can be improved by almost 200% over three months using PNF stretching as compared with static (slow) or ballistic (bouncing) stretching.

PNF involves a static stretch followed by a strong isometric contraction of a muscle against an immovable resistance (e.g. a partner). The Golgi's tendon organ is stimulated, eliciting the inverse stretch reflex (muscle relaxation). The muscle is then stretched further statically and the action repeated. Each isometric contraction is held for about 6 seconds (see Fig. 5.1).

For PNF stretching the following precautions should be observed:

• It should only be attempted after a total body warm-up.

• The isometric contraction should never be explosive.

• A partner should provide only resistance in the isometric phase and mild assistance in the static stretch phase.

• The isometric contraction should involve a gradual increase in effort in the first 2 seconds, which is then sustained for an additional 4 seconds.

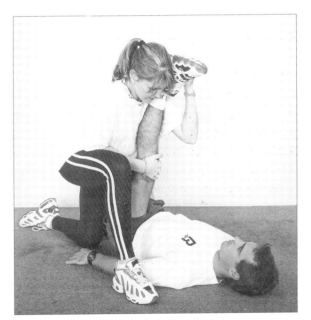

Figure 5.1: **Hamstring stretch with partner.
Start by lying on the back , raising one leg and
statically stretching it. Contract the hamstrings
isometrically against the partner for 6 seconds.
Relax them and statically stretch the hamstrings
further, and repeat the procedure.**

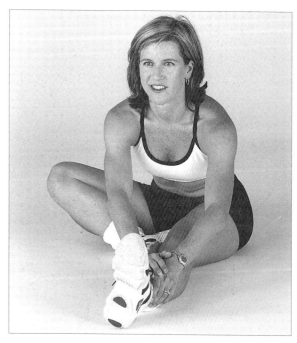

Figure 5.2: **Hamstring stretch.**

Bend one leg and place the heel close to the knee of the straight leg. With the back straight, reach towards the ankle with the hands. By holding the ankle and isometrically contracting the hamstrings and back muscles, the stretch incorporates PNF principles.

Why PNF stretching works

The PNF system is based on two fundamental principles:

1. Due to the stimulation of Golgi's tendon organ, a muscle can relax more fully after it has undergone a maximal isometric contraction.

2. A muscle becomes stronger if its antagonist is isometrically contracted immediately before stretching.

The preliminary isometric contraction makes the muscle more relaxed while it is being stretched. It also strengthens the contraction of the opposing muscles, which are used to pull the body part into a more extreme stretch position.

PNF stretching was first developed by Herman Kabat in the 1940s and was primarily used for the rehabilitation of injured muscles. It has been suggested that it works through two processes:

1. 'Irradiation', or the spread of excitation through synergistic muscle contraction,

2. 'Successive induction', which is the enhanced agonistic effort achieved after an antagonistic contraction.

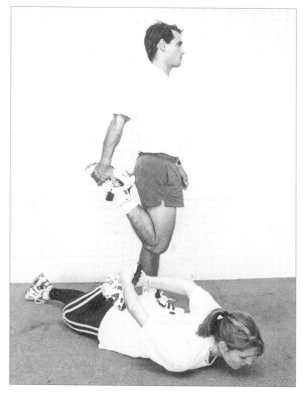

Figure 5.3: **Quadricep stretch.**

While standing or lying down pull the heel of the bent leg into the buttock. When doing this stretch it is important to keep the knees together. Again, this stretch can incorporate PNF principles.

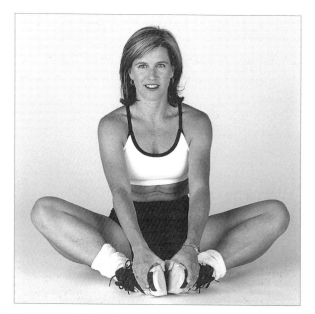

Figure 5.4: **Adductor stretch.**

Start by placing the heels together and resting the elbows on the knees. Exert pressure on the knees with the elbows for 6 seconds. Relax, then repeat the procedure with the knees wider apart.

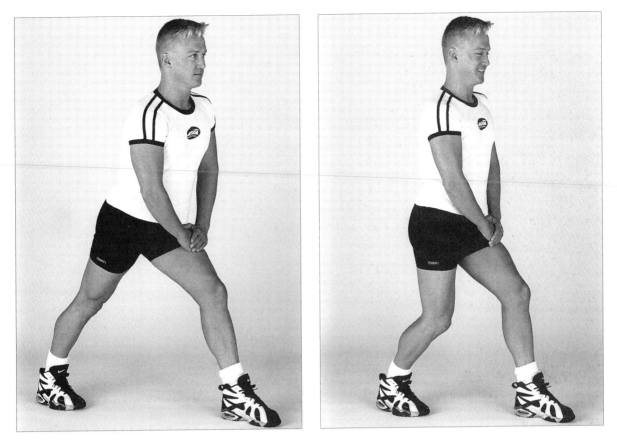

Figure 5.5: **Calf stretch.**

When stretching the calf both the gastrocnemius and soleus muscles should be stretched. To stretch the gastrocnemius the back leg is straight (above left) and to stretch the soleus it is bent (above right). Ensure that in both stretches the upper body weight is taken on the front leg.

Dr Laurence Holt from Dalhousie University in Canada has carried out research on PNF stretching. Holt compared three stretching techniques: static, ballistic and PNF stretching in increasing trunk flexion in the seated position.

After three months, the average increase in range of motion for the slow, static method was 1.7 cm, for the ballistic method slightly less than 1.7 cm, and for the PNF technique nearly 5 cm or almost three times greater than either of the other two methods.

PNF stretching is best done with a partner, although exercises can also be carried out individually (see Fig. 5.2).

Overstretching is identified by a feeling of tension or mild pain that becomes greater the longer the stretch is held. Vibrating or quivering of the muscles also suggest overstretching.

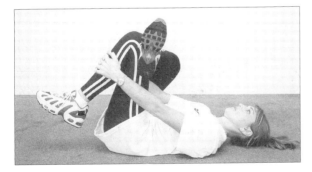

Figure 5.6: **Gluteal stretch.**

Pull the leg towards the chest. Incorporate a PNF stretch by contracting the held leg for 6 seconds, then relaxing and repeating.

Developmental stretch

A developmental stretch should follow an easy stretch. In this case the tension of the stretch is increased to a level just beyond the easy stretch. The increased distance is determined by the tension felt, and not by a specific goal. This stretch should again be held for at least 15 seconds, thereby allowing muscle fibres to stretch out slowly and stay stretched for a period of time. In the proper developmental stretch, the feeling of the stretch should decrease the longer the stretch is held, as it did with the easy stretch.

A Warning on Stretching

It should be pointed out that the field of flexibility training has only recently attracted the interest of researchers, hence there is much to learn. Meanwhile, not all authorities accept the value of stretching.

For example, US sports medicine physician Richard H. Dominguez, author of the *Complete Book of Sports Medicine*, claims stretching before exercise can cause rather than prevent injury.

According to Dominguez, runners in particular may overstretch muscles and tendons beyond a point of active control. This could cause muscle fibre damage where prior problems exist in knees or joints. Instead of excessive static stretching, Dominguez favours a warm-up of a gentle range of motion exercises, starting gradually and building up.

Critics of the Dominguez view claim that although it has some merit, it can be over-generalised. In exercise like gymnastics or floor classes where range of motion demands are great, gentle stretching is necessary, as well as a general warm-up.

Specific Flexibility Test

The following five flexibility tests require no equipment and can be used to assess flexibility on a group basis, such as in an aerobic class.

Test 1: Sit-and-reach

This is a general flexibility test for the lower back and hamstring muscle groups. Adequate flexibility in the back and hamstrings is considered very important for the prevention of lower back pain. The lower back and hamstrings are very common sites of tightness in the general population as well as in some groups of athletes. Because of its simplicity and quickness, the sit-and-reach test is the single most commonly used test for flexibility in fitness evaluations.

Procedure
- Sit on the floor with the legs out straight.
- Place the soles of the feet against a flat board.
- With the legs straight, bend forward at the hips.
- Reach forward and with the hands, try to touch the toes and then stretch past the toes.

Goals
- Not touching the toes is poor.
- Touching the toes is average.
- Reaching a hand length beyond the toes is very good.
- Reaching up to the middle of the forearm is excellent.

For more detailed comparison tables for the sit-and-reach test see Chapter 10.

Test 2: Hamstring test

The sit-and-reach test is a good overall flexibility test that measures the range of movement of a number of joints.

The following hamstring test specifically measures the suppleness of the hamstring muscles, reflected by the maximum possible angle of hip flexion.

Procedure
- Lie on the back with both legs out straight.
- Keep the lower back flat and raise one leg to the vertical position.
- A partner can stabilise the raised leg and gently push the leg to maximum hip flexion.

Goals
- Less than 90^0 at the hip is poor.
- 90^0 at the hip is acceptable.
- 105^0 at the hip is good.

Test 3: Quadriceps test

The quadriceps muscle group is a hip flexor and plays an important role in correct pelvic alignment. In addition adequate quadriceps flexibility reduces the risk of kneecap problems such as chrondromalacia patellar and patellar tendinitis.

Procedure
- Lie on the stomach with both legs out straight.
- Bend one knee so that the heel of the foot is close to the buttocks.
- Contract the abdominals to keep the hips on the floor.
- Have a partner gently push the ankle towards the buttocks.

Goals
- Heel not touching the buttock is poor.
- Heel touching the buttock is average.
- Heel touching the buttock with no resistance is good.

Test 4: Shoulder extension test

Adequate shoulder extensor flexibility is very important for allowing correct biomechanics when the arms are used in an overhead position. Inadequate flexibility can potentially contribute to shoulder injury as well as compensatory upper back injury.

Procedure
* Sit on the floor with the knees comfortably bent.
* Bring the arm (straight) forward and fully overhead.
* Throughout the movement contract the abdominals to prevent the back from arching or rotating.
* A partner can gently push the back to its maximum range of movement.

Goals
* Straight arm in front of the shoulder is poor.
* Straight arm in line with the shoulder and hip is good.
* Straight arm behind the shoulder is good.

Rules for Stretching

The following are basic principles which should be followed in any program involving stretching:

* Breathe slowly, deeply and evenly.
* Do not stretch to the point where breathing is strained.
* Do not overstretch. Go to the point where the stretch is felt but is not painful.
* Hold the stretch in a comfortable position; tension should subside as the stretch is held.
* Stretch only when the muscles are warm.
* Concentrate on relaxing the area being stretched.
* If appropriate, combine different types of stretching in one session. Avoid ballistic or bouncy stretching.
* Stretch before and after an extended exercise period.
* Hold static stretches for 15 to 30 seconds and if possible even longer.

Guidelines for Flexibility Training

The following are tips for flexibility training based on some of the limited research evidence available:
* Bouncy, jerky movements should be avoided. These can be potentially hazardous, particularly with untrained muscles.
* Stretching should progress from major joints to more specific joints. This ensures adequate support for all muscle groups involved.
* Stretching should be carried out immediately before, after and even during an active sports event. Research has shown that up to one third of the flexibility gains from stretching can be lost in half an hour of sitting still before competition, and up to two-thirds in an hour.
* Identifying the movements of the sport and training specifically in these movements should develop sport-specific flexibility.
* Flexibility training should be regular, i.e. 3–4 times a week. Noticeable increases in flexibility with training can be achieved within 2–3 weeks. Decreases can occur almost as quickly.
* If stretching is discontinued as a result of injury, qualified advice should be sought before flexibility training is recommenced.
* Stretching involving hyperextension of the lower back can often aggravate minor injuries and therefore should involve special care and attention, particularly with inexperienced exercisers.
* Pregnant women should only undertake flexibility training under supervision. During pregnancy, hormones are released which soften ligaments to make the skeletal structures of the hips and pelvis extensible for carrying an infant. This increases the hypermobility of joints, but exercises that place strain on these hypermobile joints can cause pain and chronic joint problems.
* With PNF stretching, careful attention should be paid to the correct execution of exercises. If this is not done, the results could be counter-productive.
* The optimal time for holding an isometric contraction in a PNF stretch is 6 seconds. Other static stretching can be held from 15–30 seconds.

Exercise Programming for Strength and Resistance Training

Weight training or resistance training is traditionally viewed by the community as a pastime for bodybuilders and strength athletes who wish to 'pump iron' to increase muscle size. For Fitness Instructors the area of resistance training is more far-reaching than this view. For example, an aerobic class is a form of resistance training where body weight is the resistance. Many classes now incorporate the use of dumbbells and barbells to improve muscular endurance.

Resistance training has gained acceptance with a variety of people, from the distance runner who lifts weights to maintain some upper body development or improve sports performance, to women who wish to improve muscle tone and strength outside the class environment.

The Benefits of Weight Resistance Training

There are many positive benefits of weight training, some of these are listed below. Weight training can:

- be structured to develop muscular strength, strength endurance, speed and power;
- make significant changes in body composition through increases in fat-free mass;
- improve posture;
- be structured to condition muscles specifically for sports performance;
- be used to rehabilitate muscles following injury;
- help maintain losses in muscle mass that normally occur with increased age. This helps counter the decreases that occur basal metabolic with age;
- be adapted to all fitness levels;
- increase metabolic rate through increases in muscle mass;
- help counter the decreases in metabolic rates that occur with ageing through maintenance of muscle mass.

Weight Training Terminology

Resistance training programs will vary according to the specific requirement of the program. Variations in general are based on:

Purpose	Load	% of 1 RM	Reps	Sets	Exercise Speed	Rest	Days Per Week
Strength: Advanced	heavy	85-95	2-6	1-6	slow/medium	3-5 min	2–3
Beginner	heavy	70-80	8-12	2-3	slow/medium	1-3 min	2–3
Power	medium/heavy	80-90	4-8	3-6	fast/max explosive	2-5 min	2–3
Lean Body Mass	low/medium	60-80	6-20	1-5	very slow /medium	1-2 min	2–3
Muscular Endurance	light	50-75	15-30	2-3	med	minimal	2–3

Table 6.1: **Resistance training regimes**

Repetitions (reps): the performance of a single entire exercise from the start position and back.

Sets: the number of repetitions of an exercise that can be performed to fatigue without rest.

Resistance (load): the amount of weight used in an exercise.

Repetition maximum: (RM) — or the maximum number of repetitions that can be completed with a given resistance (e.g. a 10 RM is performed when only 10 repetitions can be completed, not 9 or 11). Hence the greater the number of RM the lighter the load. The development of a particular feature of muscle performance is directly related to the load used (e.g. for improvements in strength a 3–6 RM should be used, whereas for muscular endurance a 12–15 RM should be used). The 1 RM method is based on a percentage of the maximum load that can be lifted in 1 repetition. For example, if a client's 1 RM is 100 kg then an 80% load would be 80 kg. This method should only be used with experienced lifters and should be restricted to determining loads for compound exercises. Some exercises require care in using RM loading, due to possible injury. A classic example is the military press, which can place enormous stress on the lower back if the correct technique is not used.

Rest: is necessary for the re-growth of muscle tissue after overload. Also, rest periods are dependent on the energy systems the person wishes to stress and the specific purpose for which the training is being undertaken.

Uses of Resistance Training

Resistance training can be used for one or more of the following purposes:

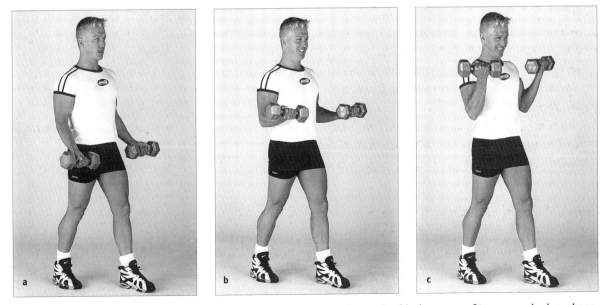

Figure 6.1: **The Biceps Curl — a. Strong commencement phase — b. Weak mid phase — c. Strong conclusion phase.**

* to increase strength, which is the ability to exert force;
* to improve power — the ability to exert force in a short period of time;
* to increase lean body tissue — this refers to the hypertrophy of muscle to increase body size. Often referred to as muscle bulk;
* to improve muscular endurance — the capacity of a muscle or muscle group to keep contracting efficiently over extended periods of time.

Resistance training regimes for strength, power, lean body mass and muscular endurance are summarised in Table 6.1. In certain circumstances a combination of these can be carried out, i.e. strength and muscle endurance.

Forms of Resistance Training

There are three general forms of resistance training. Constant resistance, variable resistance and accommodating resistance.

1. Constant resistance

When using constant resistance equipment, the level of effort changes throughout the range of motion. As the angle of pull varies, the weight lifted either feels heavier (sometimes referred to as the sticking point) or lighter depending on the angle of the joint. An example is the biceps curl, where the sticking point occurs between 800 and 1000 of elbow flexion (see Figure 6.1). It is easier to curl the bar at the beginning and end of the movement than at the midpoint. Examples of constant resis-

tance training include free weights (barbells and dumbbells), the lifter's own body weight (chins and dips) and some of the older style pin-loaded weight machines.

2. Variable resistance

Variable resistance equipment compensates for the changes in leverage through a joint's range of motion. This equipment relates the body's leverage with the machine; it attempts to exert maximum intensity on the muscles over the complete range of motion. Variable resistance equipment imposes an increasing load throughout the range of movement of the joint. This is accomplished through changing the relationship of the fulcrum and the lever arm in the weight machine as the exercise progresses.

3. Accommodating resistance

By controlling the speed of movement, it is possible to considerably improve the overload through the entire range of movement. Using hydraulic systems, air systems and clutch plates in tandem with flywheels does this. Accommodating resistance devices allows maximum force to be applied against the resistance through the entire range of motion. Most of these accommodating resistance devices can also be adjusted to infinite gradations of speed, ranging from very fast to very slow.

Types of Muscle Contraction

There are three main types of muscle contraction of interest to the weight trainer:

RATING THE EFFECTS OF EQUIPMENT TYPES ON SELECTED TRAINING GOALS ON SCALE OF 1 TO 10						
	Dumbbells & Barbells	Constant Resistance Machines	Cam Machines	Lever Machines	Hydraulic Machines	Clutch & Flywheel Machines
Increased muscle size	10	8	7	7	5	5
Increased muscle strength	10	8	7	7	5	7
Increased explosive power	9	8	7	7	10	10
Enhanced sport-specific movement	9	7	5	5	5	8
Enhanced sport skills (velocity/acceleration)	9	6	5	4	7	7
Quality of overload throughout the entire exercise set	6	6	7	7	6	7
Quality of muscular isolation	10	9	8	8	8	9
Total effectiveness score	73	59	50	52	52	60

Table 6.2: **The effectiveness of the different systems in resistance training.**

	COMPARATIVE RATING		
Criterion	Isokinetic	Isometric	Isotonic
Rate of strength gain	Excellent	Poor	Good
Rate of endurance gain	Excellent	Poor	Good
Strength gain over range of motion	Excellent	Poor	Good
Time per training session	Good	Excellent	Poor
Expense	Poor	Excellent	Good
Ease of performance	Good	Excellent	Poor
Ease of progress assessment	Poor	Good	Excellent
Adaptability to specific movements	Good	Poor	Excellent
Least possibility of muscle soreness	Excellent	Good	Poor
Least possibility of injury	Excellent	Good	Poor
Skill improvement	Excellent	Poor	Good

Table 6.3: **Summary of advantages and disadvantages of the three most common types of resistance training programs.**

1. Isometric training

The term isometric comes from the Greek *isometrikos* meaning literally 'the same length' or 'no change in length'. Isometric (or static) exercises are those done where a muscle develops tension without changing length. In fact, the muscle does shorten internally during an isometric contraction, but a contraction of the antagonist muscle or the resistance of an immovable object counters this.

Isometrics are useful for developing strength in weak spots and for increasing strength and preventing injury at the limits of the range of motion. Isometrics are particularly useful for sports such as downhill skiing, judo, gymnastics and windsurfing, where a position may have to be held for some time.

Although isometric training received quite a deal of attention in the 1950s and 1960s it is rarely practised today unless it is included with other weight training techniques. Strength increases associated with isometric training are specific to the joint angle at which the training is performed, so a full range of motion training effect using this method is impractical. The static nature of isometric training offers little benefit to most sports, which are dynamic in nature.

Some problems associated with isometric training include: minimal training of the neuromuscular system; progress is difficult to assess and hence motivation to keep training may be hard to attain; and isometric contractions produce significantly higher systolic and diastolic blood pressures.

Functional isometric training for various sports can be carried out using weights or movable resistance where an isometric contraction is combined with an isotonic movement. For example, the following exercises with weights can be made isometric by holding the resistance at the joint angle specified:

Exercise	Joint angle
Bench press	Elbow joint at 90°
Arm curls	Elbow joint at 90°
Heel raises	Foot at 135°
Dead lift	Knee joint at 135°

2. Isotonic training

The term 'isotonic' means of 'equal tension'. It implies that the muscle develops a certain tension or force in lifting and lowering a load. In fact, the force developed by the muscle is variable, depending on the position of the lever-arm at the joint.

There are two types of isotonic contractions: concentric and eccentric contractions.

i)   A concentric contraction is often referred to as a positive contraction. It is a contraction where the muscle develops tension when shortening. For example, the upward phase of the biceps curl while the biceps are shortening is a concentric contraction.

ii) An eccentric contraction is often referred to as a negative contraction. It is a contraction where the muscle develops tension while lengthening. For example, when the biceps lengthen under load during the downward phase of the biceps curl an eccentric contraction occurs. Put simply, the eccentric phase occurs when the muscle is acting as a brake against the force of gravity, i.e. when lowering a weight.

In the bench press exercise the triceps and pectorals contract eccentrically in the descent phase and then contract concentrically to bring the bar back to the starting position (Fig. 6.2).

In order to get the greatest benefit out of the eccentric contraction, the muscle must work against gravity. As a general rule the eccentric phase should take twice as long as the concentric phase, i.e. if the concentric phase takes 2 seconds the eccentric should take 4 seconds.

Isotonic training with weights was developed in the late 1940s using the concept of Repetition Maximum (RM) for determining the amount of weight used. An RM is defined as the maximal load a muscle or muscle group can lift a given number of times before fatiguing. For years it has been thought that strength could be improved only by using heavy resistance with low repetitions and that conversely, endurance could be enhanced by using light resistance with high repetitions. Recent studies have shown, however, that there is a good deal of carry-over from one type of training to another, even though the basic principle may still apply.

3. Isokinetic training

An isokinetic contraction is one in which maximal tension is developed throughout the full range of movement at a constant rotational speed. This requires special equipment in which speed of the movement is kept constant through the full range of the movement regardless of the tension applied.

Isokinetic training is relatively new and has therefore not yet been extensively evaluated scientifically. Research that has been carried out has shown significant strength gains. But in comparison with other isotonic devices the gains are relative to the type of equipment used for evaluation. For example, athletes trained on isokinetic machines develop greater increases in strength than athletes trained isotonically, if the measure of strength is isokinetic. If the measure is isotonic, the opposite is true.

Isokinetic training is particularly useful in the rehabilitation of injury and in specific sports training which requires maximal power output throughout the full range of motion at given speed.

Modern Resistance Training Systems

Hydraulic equipment

Hydraulic equipment varies the resistance relative to the speed of movement throughout the range of motion. This system, using hydraulic cylinders, incorporates both isotonic and isokinetic principles. The cylinders have 1–6 settings allowing for changes in resistance. A setting of 1 allows for a large aperture between the cylinders, which provides light resistance. Conversely, a setting of 6 allows for a small aperture resulting in a greater resistance.

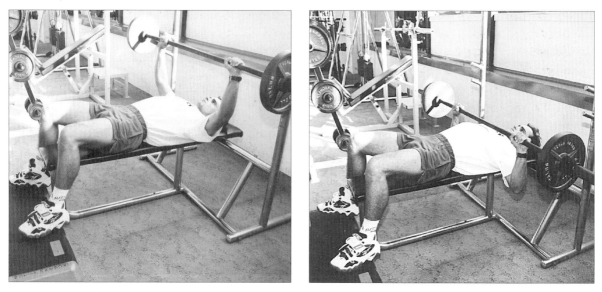

Figure 6.2: **The bench press** (above). **The upward phase** (left) **is concentric; the downward phase** (right), **eccentric.**

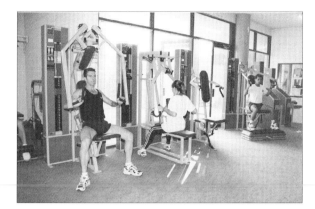

Figure 6.3: **Modern resistance training —
the Medex RT system.**

The action of the hydraulic cylinders used provide the lifter with a double concentric movement, allowing for two antagonistic movements to be completed using one piece of equipment.

Variable resistance isotonic

The heart of the Nautilus system is the cam, which is an 'off-round' wheel with a non-central axis of rotation shaped like a nautilus shell.

The radius of the Nautilus cam changes as it turns. This acts to automatically vary the load to accommodate the weak and strong phases of the lifting stroke.

Dynamic variable resistance (DVR) isotonic

DVR machines consist of a variety of pin-loaded weight stations designed using pulleys and guide rails. Universal's DVR machines vary resistance to accommodate changes in biomechanical advantage to ensure maximum muscular effort throughout the full range of movement. A visual scale on the lever arm shows the percentage of increase of resistance driving the lifting stroke.

Air pressure

Pressurised pneumatic cylinders with compressed air create the resistance in this system. A pressure regulator located within easy reach of the trainee is used to vary air pressure so that the resistance can be varied. This system allows for both concentric and eccentric contraction over the full range of movement. As air is compressed within the cylinder the pressure increases, thus increasing the force output on the lifter.

Modern Techniques of Overload

The progressive overload principle is one of the most fundamental and important tenets of muscle physiology. It states that to elicit improvements in muscle size, strength or endurance, the muscle must be placed under stress levels greater than it was previously used to and in a way specific to the required physiological outcomes (Fig. 6.4). This can be achieved by either:

- increasing the resistance or weight load;
- increasing the number of repetitions;
- increasing the speed of contraction;
- increasing the volume of the workout (sets, exercises);
- decreasing the rest periods (up to a point) between sets.

More esoteric overloading techniques, sometimes based on unclear physiological principles, have been used for years, particularly by bodybuilders and sports trainers. In fact, this is one aspect of resistance training where the practice has often preceded the theory.

It is clear that individuality has to be taken into consideration in evaluating overloading practices. Where some individuals respond well to some overloading techniques, others may not. Hence it is important for the fitness instructor to know the range of techniques available. The following is a list of overload techniques gathered from sports training and bodybuilding practices.

1. Blitzing: This is the practice of bombarding a muscle or muscle group on any one training day. This can take the form of several exercises aimed at working the muscle from different angles.

2. Forced repetitions: These require a partner or 'spotter' so that assistance can be given in that part of the movement where biomechanical advantage is least (the sticking point). This then means a heavier weight can be lifted through the full range of movement.

For example, in the arm curl motion a 'sticking point' is reached about where the elbows are at right angles. If assistance is given through this point, a heavier weight can be used through the full range of motion.

When spotting a lifter, whether it be for forced reps or just during a normal set, the spotter should:

- concentrate throughout the lift;
- check that the bar is loaded correctly;
- check that weights are secured by using collars;
- determine what signals to use;
- determine how many reps are to be attempted;
- always check the lifter's form;
- encourage the lifter.

Shoulders	Dumbell lateral raise
	Upright row
Chest	Dumbell flyes
	Bench press
Thighs	Leg extension
	Squats
Back	Lat pulldown
	Seated row
Biceps	Preacher curl
	Narrow grip chin up
Triceps	Pressdown
	Dips

3. Cheating: This is a technique recommended only for experienced weight trainers, where auxiliary muscles are used to assist a prime mover in a movement. For example, in arm curls the trunk is bent forward slightly enabling the contraction of the back muscles to assist the lifter to lift a heavier weight through the weakest point of the movement. This means a heavier weight can be used and the muscle is thus overloaded through the strong phases of the movement.

When cheating, remember to use gentle body motions to assist lifting the weight to the finished position. Never snap the weight through its range of motion.

4. Negative repetitions: These capitalise on the fact that strength and bulk improvements in muscle are aided by exaggerated eccentric (lowering) contractions of the muscle. In a negative repetition the weight is only lowered, enabling more weight to be used to overstress the muscle eccentrically. Spotters are required to lift the weight for the lifter so that it can then be lowered.

An example of negative repetitions would be where the weight is lowered to the chest slowly in the bench press and then returned to the rack by the spotters so the action can be repeated.

5. Pre-exhaustion: This is where a muscle is isolated in an exercise and fatigued before being co-opted for further work in a compound exercise which immediately follows.

The second or compound exercise enables the muscle previously exhausted to continue working because it is aided by synergist muscles.

An example of a complete pre-exhaust workout is as follows:

6. Rest pause: This is a technique practised by bodybuilders for increasing intensity of effort. It is done by overloading a muscle such that only 1 RM can be carried out and a pause is necessary (perhaps 10 seconds) before it can be done again and again, over a set number of repetitions.

This is a high-intensity technique that should be carried out only by experienced lifters.

7. Up and down the rack: This is a principle similar to pyramiding, except that weights from light to heavy gradations are arranged on a weight rack and exercises carried out with each of these, with weight increasing and then decreasing, until exhaustion.

8. Pyramid training: This refers to the practice of increasing resistance step by step over sets or repetitions. It allows the person to start easily, build up to a peak and then taper off. The resistance is increased step by step over a number of sets then the load is decreased when the peak is reached (Table 6.4).

Sets	Weight	Reps
1	50 kg	20
2	60 kg	12
3	65 kg	8
4	70 kg	4
5	60 kg	max
6	50 kg	max

Table 6.4: **The squat workout — pyramid style.**

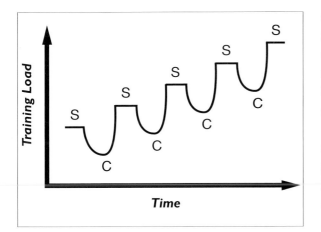

Figure 6.4: **Progressive overload — resistance training should follow the concept of progressive overload. 'S' indicates the training stimulus which is increased progressively. 'C' demonstrates performance improvement in response to training.**

9. Super-sets: Can be categorised into two distinct, but similar types of programs. One program targets the agonist and antagonist of the same body part. For example, arm curls immediately followed by tricep extensions.

The second and more common type of super-setting, uses one set of two exercises in rapid succession for the same muscle group or body part, with no rest between the sets. An example would be completing a set of 10 shoulder press exercises, followed immediately by a set of 10 side (lateral) raises. The basis of this technique is to use a compound exercise followed immediately by an isolation exercise. If the reverse order were performed then the prime mover, in the isolation exercise, would fatigue. The assisting muscles in the compound exercise would then play a more dominant role thereby reducing the load on the prime mover (see Pre-exhaustion).

Super-setting is a very high intensity overload technique. Therefore, it should not be the sole training technique utilised for all muscle groups within a training period. Instead the instructor should only target a single muscle or muscle group for super-setting in any given workout. An alternative is to target a number of muscles or muscle groups for super-setting in a single workout every 3 to 4 weeks. For example, a client who trains 3 times per week (Monday, Wednesday, Friday) could, above and beyond their normal program, super-set the chest on Monday, the shoulders on Wednesday

and the back on Friday. The following week the emphasis could switch to the legs by super-setting the quadriceps on Monday, hamstrings on Wednesday and calves on Friday. This whole process can then be repeated following a 3–4 week recovery while maintaining the normal program.

Table 6.8 lists a series of exercises that be can be used to super-set most of the major muscles or muscle groups. Option 1 details traditional compound and isolation exercises while Option 2 provides alternative exercises for the same muscle/muscle group.

- Tri-sets consist of three exercises for the same body part. The exercises can include different muscle groups and are normally performed with a minimal amount of rest betwen exercises and sets. Normally three sets of each exercise are performed. An example of a tri-set for the same body part is:
  Dumbbell bent over raises
  Press behind neck
  Dumbbell lateral raises
- Giant sets are super-sets with more than two exercises carried out without rest in between. Giant sets are used for the same body part, e.g. the chest, using bench press followed by:
  'Pec' dec
  Incline dumbbell press
  Dumbbell flyes.

10. Hybrid exercise/compound repetitions: This method involves the use of several joints of the body moving through a greater range of motion than is normal with single exercises. Thus, instead of carrying out three or four exercises in a circuit, they can all be done in the one repetition. For example, the power clean could be followed by a front squat, then a push press, then an overhead squat, then finish by lowering the bar to chest and placing it on the ground.

11. Triple drop: For many years bodybuilders and other athletes have used the method of dropping or reducing the level of resistance (weight) during a set of repetitions to work a muscle area as thoroughly as possible. This is done by choosing a weight on a barbell, dumbbell or machine that permits the user to perform only three or four repetitions. When failure occurs, assistants remove only enough weight (usually 10%) to allow continuation of the exercise for another three or four repetitions. This procedure is repeated three times or until the muscle group is worked to a point of complete failure.

12. Single set system: This refers to the performance of each exercise for one set. It is one of the oldest overload techniques around. In recent years it has come into vogue and is often referred to as Quality Resistance Training (QRT) or One Set to Fail. Its recent popularity is based on the fact that it is ideal for new trainers, it is time-efficient, it helps alleviate the boredom that is often experienced when completing the traditional 3-set system, it can be easily integrated into a cross training program, and it prevents congestion on equipment at peak times. When structuring a Single Set program the following should be taken into consideration:

Number of repetitions. For most individuals a repetition scheme of 8–12 is suggested.

Intensity of the set. The optimal training intensity is achieved by successive repetitions until concentric failure occurs.

Progressive overload. Each exercise should be conducted to failure, and once approximately 12 repetitions have been performed, the load should be increased by no more than 5%.

Exercise speed. An ideal movement speed for the weight is four seconds for the lifting phase (concentric), pausing momentarily, and four seconds for the lowering phase (eccentric).

Range of motion. Each exercise should be performed throughout a full range of joint movement.

Frequency of workouts. With this type of training recovery is crucial. It is recommended that a minimum of two and a maximum of three workouts be performed per week.

Machine or free weights. Both systems can be used effectively using this overload technique.

Designing Weight Training Programs

1. Building lean body mass for beginners
- Use a moderate weight, i.e. 8–12 RM.
- Select one compound and one isolation exercise per body part. For example, for the chest select the bench press followed by the 'pec dec'.
- Perform 2–3 sets of the 8–12 RM for each exercise in every workout. When more than 12 reps can be completed in the final set increase the weight used 2–5%. Initially only use 1 set of each exercise for the first 2–4 weeks.
- Exercise three days per week with a rest day in between each workout.

2. Building lean body mass for intermediate to advanced
- Vary the load of the weights used. For example, alternate one heavy session of 4–6 RM with a medium session of 8–12 RM or use a pyramid-type protocol. These sessions should be alternated in a split workout (4 days a week).
- Increase the number of exercises to work the muscles from a variety of angles.
- Increase the total number of sets (2–5) per exercise.
- Allow adequate recuperation time, at least 1 rest day for smaller muscle groups and 2 days for larger muscle groups.

3. Developing a strength training program
- Most authorities suggest that the resistance used should be greater than 80% of 1 RM.
- Use around 3–6 sets of less than 6 repetitions.

Checklist for programming resistance training
- Determine goals.
- Select training regime.
- Select exercises.
- Select training method.
- Select techniques of overload.
- Teach correct form.
- Evaluate progress.

- Allow adequate recuperation time, at least 1 rest day for smaller muscle groups and 2 days for larger muscle groups.
- Use mostly compound movements and select 2–4 exercises per body part.
- Where possible incorporate periodisation (see p.66) into the strength program.
- Use exercises that are event-specific when programming for enhanced sports performance.

Sports trainers suggest the following program to increase strength after a general warm-up is performed:

Load   90–95% of 1 RM
Reps   2–3
Sets   2–3
Rest   9–10 secs between reps 4–6 mins between sets.

This style of training can only be maintained for periods of about 6 weeks and is often interspersed with a muscle hypertrophy program such as:

Load   75–80% of 1 RM
Reps   8–12
Sets   2–3
Rest   1.5–2 mins between sets.

Instructors should note that the above strength programs are only recommended for experienced resistance trainers.

4. Developing speed or explosive strength

Moving a heavy external resistance as quickly as possible can develop explosive strength. Variations in the percentage of the 1 RM used in combination with speed of contraction dictate the training adaptations for these two categories.

An example of a speed/strength program is as follows:

Load   30–70% 1 RM
Reps   6–8 with high velocity
Sets   2–3 repeated 2–3 times
Rest   9–10 secs between reps
         4–6 mins between sets
         8–10 mins between sequences.

In recent years a form of explosive training called plyometrics, which is used for developing explosive speed, has come into vogue. Plyometric exercises utilise the elastic forces that are generated while a muscle undergoes pre-stretch during the eccentric phase. This is followed by a rapid concentric contraction of the same muscles.

The most common plyometrics exercise is the depth jump, where the person stands on a box up to 1 metre high, then jumps off the box and lands on the balls of the feet. This is followed by an explosive vertical jump. To develop optimal speed and strength the time on the ground should be minimal: if too long is spent on the ground the elastic tension developed during the eccentric contraction will be lost into the ground instead of being converted to concentric force (see Figure 6.5).

Plyometric exercises can be planned using: jumps, medicine ball throws, handstand jumps and clap pushups. In fact the only limiting factor to developing plyometric exercises is the instructor's imagination.

Plyometric exercise is a high-stress activity and should only be prescribed for advanced exercisers with an adequate strength base.

5. Developing muscular endurance

Muscular endurance refers to tolerance against fatigue following high repetition work. The aim in training for muscular endurance is to maintain somewhat higher tension in the muscles than they are normally accustomed to.

An example of a strength endurance program is as follows:

Load   60–80% 1RM
Reps   15–25 (to muscle failure)
Sets   2–3
Rests   Gradually reduced between sets from 90 to
         30 seconds.

Circuit training is an ideal method of training muscular endurance (see Chapter 4) as the manipulation of the load and rest periods can be adapted to the specific needs of each individual.

6. Toning program

The basic guidelines for developing a toning program are:

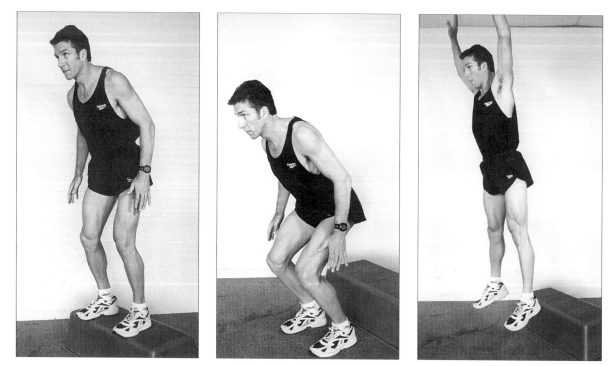

Figure 6.5: **The depth jump (plyometrics).**

- 🏃 light to moderate weight;
- 🏃 1–2 sets per exercise;
- 🏃 2–3 exercises per body part;
- 🏃 use mainly compound movements;
- 🏃 use a circuit structure;
- 🏃 program 3 sessions per week.

7. Circuit training with weights

Research on traditional weight training programs show that it doesn't produce any significant cardiovascular training effect. Although individual exercises may be strenuous, the amount of time devoted to the exercises *per se* is usually short. The rate of oxygen consumed has been estimated to be roughly the equivalent of walking at 6 km per hour pace, gardening or swimming at a slow speed. This means that such exercise would be of little value as the major component of a body fat reduction or cardiovascular conditioning program.

It is possible to achieve a cardiovascular benefit by incorporating resistance exercises into an aerobic circuit (see Chapter 4). In the fitness centre situation this provides an opportunity for resistance training to be performed on either an individual or group basis, using traditional free weights or the modern weight training systems mentioned above.

Variations Training

Periodisation

The term periodisation refers to dividing the training program into a number of training periods that vary in their purpose depending on the goals of the client.

The rationale behind periodisation is that there are three phases of the body's adaptation when it is confronted with a stress stimulus. These are:

1. Shock: when the body is confronted with a new training stimulus, soreness develops and performance actually decreases.

2. Adaptation to the stimulus: the body adapts to the new training stimulus and performance increases.

3. Staleness: the body has adapted to the stimulus and adaptations are no longer taking place.

There are many forms of periodisation. One technique used by resistance trainers is simply to vary the intensity of their lifts over a weekly period:

Weeks	1–2	3–4	5–6	7–8	9–10	11–12
Reps	10–12	4–6	8–10	3–5	6–8	2–3
Sets	3	5	4	5	4	6
Intensity*	70–75%	82–88%	75–78%	85–90%	80–85%	90–95%
Volume**	30–36	20–30	32–40	15–25	24–32	12–18

* Intensity refers to the percentage of 1RM being lifted in a workout.

** Volume can be defined as the total number of repetitions performed in a workout or the total amount of weight lifted in a workout (sets x reps x load).

Table 6.6: **An example of periodisation**

Phase	Hypertrophy	Basic Strength	Strength and power	Peaking* or maintenance
Sets	3–5	3–5	3–5	1–3
Reps	8–20	2–6	2–3	1–3
Days/week	3–4	3–5	4–6	1–5
Times/day	1–3	1–3	1–2	1
Intensity cycle (weeks) **	2–3/1	2–4/1	2–3/1	–
Intensity	low	high	high to low	Very high
Volume	high	Moderate to high	low	very low

* Peaking for sports with a definite climax, or maintenance for sports with a long season such as football.

** Ratio of number of heavy training weeks to light training weeks.

Table 6.7: **A periodised model for resistance training.**

Muscles	Option 1 Compound	Option 1 Isolation	Option 2 Compound	Option 2 Isolation
Pectoralis major	Supine bench press	Supine flyes	Incline bench press	Pec deck
Latissimus dorsi	Lat pull down	Bent over row	Wide grip chin up (barbell)	Dumbbell pullover
Deltoids	Shoulder press	Dumbbell raise 1. Anterior 2. Lateral 3. Posterior	Upright row	Cable work
Triceps	Dips	Triceps cable pushdown	Close grip bench-press	Overhead single arm triceps extensions (dumbbell)
Biceps	Close grip chin ups	Isolation curls (dumbbells)	Dumbbell curls with shoulder flexion	Preacher curls
Quadriceps	Squat (front, back, smith machine)	Leg extension	Leg press	
Gluteus maximus	Squat	Hip extension	Lunges	
Hamstrings	Stiff legged dead lifts	Leg curl	Lunges	
Calves	Standing barbell toe raise	Seated calf raise		
Lower back	Barbell clean	Back extension		

Table 6.8: **Selection of exercises.**

Workout 1	Heavy (3–5 RM)
Workout 2	Light (12–15 RM)
Workout 3	Medium (8–10 RM)

A second technique, for highly motivated resistance trainers, is to work at 100% intensity for the three workouts but to change the exercise to fit the heavy-light-medium format. For example, a trainer may select three exercises that overload the shoulder girdle (bench press, military press and incline press) and vary the weight to suit each exercise.

A third technique used by athletes is to divide the training year into a preparation period (pre-season), a competition period (in season), and a transition period (active rest). The preparation phase can be further subdivided into general and specific preparation periods, and the competition phase can be broken down into an early competition phase and a main competition phase. The transition period is normally a period of 4–5 weeks of rest and recovery (*Better Coaching — Advanced Coach's Manual*, Australian Coaching Council, 1991).

The underlying concept of periodisation is the use of training cycles. This means that the major training phases are divided into smaller cycles called macrocycles and microcycles. Macrocycles are periods of 3–5 weeks (monthly) while microcycles are 7–10 days (weekly) in length. There are usually 3–5 microcycles per macrocycle. Microcycles are further divided up into daily or twice daily routines (*Better Coaching*, 1991).

A popular periodisation model follows a linear intensification approach to strength development (Table 6.7).

🏃 Peaking for sports with a definite climax, or maintenance for sports with a long season such as football.

🏃 Ratio of the number of heavy training weeks to light training weeks.

Another approach to periodisation is alternating moderate training between more intense training in two-weekly training blocks, as demonstrated in Table 6.6.

Frequency of workout

The amount of recovery between workouts should be dependent on the recovery ability of the individual. Traditionally three workouts per week (Mon–Wed–Fri) is considered to be optimal.

The split routine

With more experienced lifters it is not practical to use the traditional three workouts per week schedule, as the training sessions would be far too long. The split routine overcomes this problem by dividing the training session into body parts. The most common form is the four-day per week split, also called the 'push and pull' workout. This is as follows:

🏃 Pushing movements are done on Mondays and Thursdays, emphasising chest, shoulders and triceps.

🏃 Pulling movements are done on Tuesdays and Fridays, emphasising legs, back and biceps.

There are many other variations of the split routine, but with most there is a definite risk of overtraining due to the amount and intensity of work that can be done in each training session.

Classification and Choice of Exercise

1. Isolation exercises: These usually isolate a single specific muscle across one joint; for example, dumbbell lateral raise, pec flyes and concentration curl.

2. Compound exercises: These exercises involve the use of many muscles and joints to produce movement; for example, bench press, squat and power clean.

Muscle Analysis and Exercise Selection

Good exercise selection is fundamental to achieving the desired goals from a resistance training program. The first priority is to identify the joints and primary muscles that move them when a particular movement is performed. A general three-step model for identification of prime mover muscles follows:

1. Identify all moving joints.
2. Identify all muscles that cross those joints.
3. Of the muscles that cross the joint, identify those with the most mechanically effective line-of-pull in relation to the load.

Using this simple three-step approach you can ensure that the exercises selected are appropriate for the muscle groups you wish to train. Tables 6.9 through to Table 6.16 analyse various major muscles including: pectoralis major, deltoid, biceps brachii, latissimus dorsi, rhomboids, gluteus maximus, biceps femoris and rectus femoris.

Safety Precautions in Resistance Training

1. When lifting weights from the floor, bench or table:
   - Stand with the feet parallel, shoulder width apart, and close to the bar.
   - Lower the hips by flexing the knees.
   - Maintain a straight back, held as vertical as possible.
   - Keep the head up.
   - Lift the weight by extending or straightening the legs.

2. Before beginning each exercise, be sure the feet are properly positioned, the pelvis is stabilised and the hands gripping the bar are an equal distance from each end of the bar.

3. Always wipe the benches down after use and return the weights to their racks. Always dismantle weights after use, e.g. the squat bar or the bench press bar.

4. Watch for frayed cables or loose collars on bars.

5. When lifting weights participants should:
   - be familiar with the equipment they wish to use;
   - use the correct lifting techniques;
   - know their limits;
   - never drop the weights after use;
   - grip the weight correctly prior to the lift;
   - load and unload the equipment correctly.

Spotting

In all resistance programs, proper spotting is necessary to ensure the safety of the exerciser. The primary role of the spotter is to assist the client with the exercise. In order to do this the spotter should:

- be strong enough to assist the client if need be;
- understand the proper technique for the lift;
- provide the correct verbal cues for the lift;
- know the correct spotting position for each lift;
- understand spotting etiquette (e.g. where to stand when the client is on his or her back, and ask permission prior to touching the client).

Choosing the Best Equipment

When considering weight training, there is a variety of machines and training systems available. While the manufacturers of each often claim special advantages, no one machine system caters for all contingencies; they all have their advantages and disadvantages. In addition, it is not uncommon to hear arguments supporting the use of machine weight training in preference to free weights, and vice versa. Below are some benefits of both free weights and machine systems.

Advantages of free weights

Specific transfer of training: This a key aspect of strength and fitness development for sports. It has been suggested that when using free weights the individual's sport-specific pattern of motor unit recruitment can be stimulated more closely than when using machine systems. This is because the freely moving bar is not being 'guided' or otherwise restrained as it is with machine systems. This results in a greater transfer of training from the weights room to the actual playing field.

Joint strength: The free weight user has to balance the resistance rather than be guided by machinery, which may be an aid in developing joint strength. Bill Star, the University of Hawaii strength coach says, 'As a football player takes a loaded barbell off the bench press stand, he must steady the bar before lowering it to the chest. The controlling action builds tendon and ligament strength in the wrist, elbow and shoulder joints.'

Muscle synergism: In normal movements, a number of 'synergist' or supporting muscles aid the prime mover. Many exercise machines, however, are constructed to isolate one or a limited number of muscles

| Targeted muscle (prime mover): | Pectoralis major |
| Antagonist: | Rhomboids and lower trapezius |

Pectoralis major

Palpation:	Broad area of chest region between the clavicle and sixth rib.
Origin:	Anterior border of the clavicle, the whole length of the sternum and the cartilages of the first 6 ribs.
Insertion:	Outer lip of the intertubercular groove of the humerus.
Muscle action:	Shoulder flexion — draws the arm forward and upward from the side. True horizontal adduction — draws the arm from the side horizontal position to the front horizontal position. Inward rotation of the humerus.
Sports action:	Used powerfully in push-ups, most throwing activities, racket sports, gymnastics and most forward movements of the humerus.
Kinesiological analysis:	This muscle is commonly divided into two parts. The clavicular portion lies close to the anterior deltoid and works with it in flexion and horizontal adduction of the humerus. The sternal portion acts only in downward and forward movements of the arm.

Muscles that assist the prime mover:

Coracobrachialis	Origin:	Coracoid process of the scapula.
	Insertion:	Inner surface of humerus opposite deltoid attachment.
Anterior deltoid	Origin:	Anterior border of the clavicle and acromion process.
	Insertion:	In front of the head of the humerus.
Triceps brachii	Origin:	Lateral and medial head — humerus. Long head — scapula.
	Insertion:	Olecranon process of the ulna.

Common exercise — **The Flat Bench Dumbbell Flye incorporates the pectoralis major's normal action.**

Exercise technique	i)	Lie on a flat bench, feet on the end of the bench.
	ii)	Lower back should be pressed into the bench.
	iii)	With arms extended raise the dumbbells directly above sternum.
	iv)	Palms should be facing each other and elbows slightly bent.
	v)	While ensuring the arms are in line, lower them in an arc motion.
	vi)	To get a complete stretch on the pectoralis, lower the arms to a point where the hands are in line with the shoulders.
	vii)	Return to the starting position through the same arc until the dumbbells lightly touch at the top.

Exercise variations:

| Free weights | Bench press, incline or decline bench press |
| Machine systems | pec dec, cable cross over, bench press machine |

Table 6.9: Pectoralis major.

Targeted muscle (prime mover):	Biceps brachii
Antagonist:	Triceps brachii

Biceps brachii

Palpation:	Anterior aspect of the humerus.
Origin:	Two heads — top of the coracoid process and upper lip of the glenoid fossa of the scapula.
Insertion:	Tuberosity of the radius.
Muscle action:	Flexion of the arm at the elbow. Supination of the forearm and weak shoulder flexion.
Sports action:	Used when climbing, chinning or raising the body to bar in gymnastics and all activities that involve pulling something to the body.
Kinesiological analysis:	The biceps is a two-headed type of muscle. It is the primary muscle involved in flexion of the elbow joint, but also acts during flexion at the shoulder joint. Maximum strength is obtained when the forearm is supinate.

Muscles that assist the prime mover:

Brachialis	Origin:	Lower half of the anterior portion of the humerus.
	Insertion:	Tuberosity of the ulna and coronoid process of the ulna.
Brachioradialis	Origin:	Lower two thirds of the outer ridge of humerus.
	Insertion:	Lateral side of base of styloid process of radius.
Deltoid	Origin:	Anterior border of clavicle, acromion process, spine of scapula.
	Insertion:	In front of the head of the humerus.

Common exercise	**The Biceps Curl effectively isolates the biceps brachii.**	
Exercise technique	i)	Start with feet shoulder width apart and hold the bar in a supinated grip.
	ii)	Arms straight and elbows touching the sides of the body.
	iii)	Move the bar upwards in an arc, while keeping the elbows stationary and to the sides.
	iv)	Bring the bar as high to the chest as the movement will allow.
	v)	Keep the elbows behind the bar at all times.
	vi)	Do not lean back to assist in any part of the movement.
	vii)	The biceps plays a small role in shoulder flexion — in order to overload the muscle completely raise the elbows at the top of the curl.
	viii)	Slowly lower the bar to the full elbow extension position.

Exercise variations:

Free weights	Incline dumbbell Biceps Curl, Standing Easy-Curl Bar, Preacher Curl
Machine systems	Universal Machine Standing Barbell Curl, Hydra Gym Biceps Machine, Nautilus Biceps Curl

Table 6.10: **Biceps brachii.**

| Targeted muscle (prime mover): | Deltoid |
| Antagonist: | Latissimus dorsi |

Deltoids

Palpation:	Over the head of the humerus from the anterior to the posterior side.
Origin:	Front outer third of the clavicle, border of the acromion and lower edge of the spine of the scapula.
Insertion:	Tubercle on the middle outer surface of humerus.
Muscle action:	True abduction — entire muscle. Shoulder flexion, horizontal adduction and inward rotation — anterior fibres. Shoulder extension, outward rotation and horizontal abduction — posterior fibres.
Sports action:	The combination of shoulder joint abduction, flexion and extension is used in sports that require hitting such as tennis and baseball, also shooting sports, which require the arms to be elevated for long periods.
Kinesiological analysis:	The deltoid is a powerful abductor of the humerus. In addition to raising the arm, it is frequently called upon to hold the arm in an elevated position for long periods of time. The arrangement of the fibres of the middle portion allows for a strong stabilising component.

Muscles that assist the prime mover:

Trapezius	Origin:	Base of skull, spines of 7th cervical and all thoracic vertebrae.
	Insertion:	Outer third of clavicle, top of the acromion and upper scapula.
Supraspinatus	Origin:	Inner two thirds of the supraspinatus fossa of the scapula.
	Insertion:	Top of the greater tubercle of the humerus.
Triceps brachii	Origin:	Lateral and medial head — humerus. Long head — scapula.
	Insertion:	Olecranon process of the ulna.

Common exercise — **Alternating (front/back) barbell press effectively works all three heads of the deltoid.**

Exercise technique		
	i)	Start with feet shoulder width and knees slightly bent.
	ii)	Hold a barbell in an overhand grip along the clavicles.
	iii)	Hands a little wider than shoulder width with elbows pointing down.
	iv)	Contract the abdominals to ensure the torso is erect.
	v)	Push the bar upwards until the arms are fully extended but not locked.
	vi)	Lower the bar behind the head until it touches the base of neck.
	vii)	Keep the head aligned with the spine and push the bar back up to top position, then lower to the front.

Exercise variations:

Free weights	Bent Over Row (Posterior), Push Press with Dumbbells, Incline lateral raise (Lateral)
Machine systems	Military Press (Anterior), Bent over rear-cable (Lateral), Cable Front Raise (Anterior)

Table 6.11: **Deltoid.**

Targeted muscle (prime mover):	Latissimus dorsi
Antagonist:	Deltoid

Latissimus dorsi

Palpation:	Lateral, posterior aspect of the trunk below the armpit.
Origin:	Posterior crest of the ilium, back of the sacrum and spinous processes of the lumbar and lower 6 thoracic vertebrae and lower 3 ribs.
Insertion:	Medial side of intertubercular groove of humerus.
Muscle action:	Extension — draws the arm from front to the side. Inward rotation of the arm. Horizontal abduction — draws the arm from the front to the side horizontal position. True adduction — draws the arm from the abducted side horizontal position to the side.
Sports action:	This muscle is used when climbing, in many swimming strokes, most gymnastic activities and other activities that require a pulling action using the arm.
Kinesiological analysis:	A broad sheet of muscle that covers the lower and middle portions of the back. The latissimus dorsi has a favourable angle of pull for backward and downward movement of the humerus, particularly when it is between 30° and 90°.

Muscles that assist the prime mover:

Teres major	Origin:	Lower end of the lateral border of the scapula.
	Insertion:	Upper anterior portion of the humerus.
Rhomboids	Origin:	Spinous processes of the upper thoracic vertebrae.
	Insertion:	Medial border of the scapula.
Pectoralis major	Origin:	Anterior border of the clavicle. Whole length of the sternum and cartilages of the 6 ribs.
	Insertion:	Outer lip of the intertubercular groove of the humerus.
Supraspinatus	Origin:	Inner two thirds of the supraspinatus fossa of the scapula.
	Insertion:	Top of the greater tubercle of the humerus.

Common exercise	**The Wide Lat Pulldown — to behind neck is the most common exercise for overloading this muscle.**

Exercise technique	i)	Sit with the shoulders directly under the bar.
	ii)	Grip the bar at each end (wide), palms facing forward.
	iii)	Arms fully extended, trunk erect — do not lean backwards.
	iv)	Draw the elbows downwards at a slow, moderate pace.
	v)	At the end of the movement attempt to draw the elbows together.
	vi)	The lift ends when the bar goes below the chin.
	vii)	Slowly extend the arms to maximum stretch and length.
	viii)	On the return the elbows should travel in a sideways plane.

Exercise variations:

Free weights	Chin Ups Pronated Grip, Incline Dumbbell Row, Bent-over Wide Grip Barbell Row
Machine systems	One Arm Cable Row, Narrow Grip Front Lat, Wide Grip Front Lat Pull, Pull Down — Overhand, Down — Overhand

Table 6.12: **Latissimus Dorsi.**

Targeted muscle (prime mover):	Rhomboids	
Antagonist:	**Pectoralis minor**	
Palpation:	Cannot be palpated, as it is located under trapezius muscle.	
Origin:	Spinous processes of the upper thoracic vertebrae.	
Insertion:	Medial border of the scapula.	
Muscle action:	Adduction — draws the scapula towards the spinal column with some elevation. In addition rhomboids draw the scapula in a downward rotation movement.	
Sports action:	This muscle comes into play in all movements when the arm is pulled to the rear such as in rowing, paddling, the butterfly stroke and archery.	
Kinesiological analysis:	The rhomboids comprise two muscles but functionally they are generally regarded as one. They play an important role in the maintenance of good posture.	
Muscles that assist the prime mover:		
Trapezius	Origin:	Base of the skull, cervical and thoracic spines.
	Insertion:	Posterior aspect of clavicle, scapula and acromion process.
Supraspinatus	Origin:	Supraspinous fossa of the clavicle.
	Insertion:	Top of greater tubercle of the humerus.
Deltoid (posterior)	Origin:	Inferior edge of scapula.
	Insertion:	In front of the head of the humerus.
Common exercise	**The Seated Rear Dumbell Raise (with hips flexed) is a safe and effective way of isolating the rhomboids.**	
Exercise technique	i)	Sit at the end of the bench, leaning forward with the chest resting on the thighs.
	ii)	Arms should be hanging perpendicular to the ground.
	iii)	Raise the dumbbells to the side, up to body level and continue until the forearms are parallel to the floor.
	iv)	Throughout the movement the arms should be slightly bent and at right angles to the body.
	v)	Lower slowly and repeat.
Exercise variations:		
Free weights	Bent-over Barbell Row, Bent over Dumbbell Row, Lat Pull Down	
Machine systems	Seated Cable Row, Reverse Pec Dec, Front Supported Machine Row	

Table 6.13: **Rhomboids.**

Targeted muscle (prime mover):	Gluteus maximus	
Antagonist:	**Psoas major**	
Palpation:	Wide area on the posterior surface of the pelvis.	
Origin:	Outer surface of the crest of the ilium, posterior surface of the sacrum and fascia of the lumbar area.	
Insertion:	Gluteal line of femur and iliotibial band of fascia latae.	
Muscle action:	Extension of the hip at the thigh. Outward rotation of the thigh and some leg adduction.	
Sports action:	The strong action of gluteus maximus is seen in running, hopping, skipping, cycling, rowing and jumping.	
Kinesiological analysis:	This large superficial muscle of the buttocks is a potentially powerful hip extensor. In addition, the uppermost fibres are in a position to abduct the thigh, while the lower portion of the muscle adduct it.	
Muscles that assist the prime mover:		
Biceps femoris	Origin:	Tuberosity of ischium and central line of femur — linea aspera.
	Insertion:	Head of the fibula and lateral condyle of tibia.
Semitendinosus	Origin:	Ischium
	Insertion:	Tibia
Semimembranosus	Origin:	Ischium
	Insertion:	Tibia
Common exercise	**The Lunge effectively overloads the gluteus maximus, especially in the return phase.**	
Exercise technique	i)	Barbell should be resting on the shoulders, with feet shoulder width apart.
	ii)	Grip on the bar should be wider than normal to ensure balance.
	iii)	Keep the head up and focus on a position at eye level.
	iv)	Keeping the trunk as erect as possible, step forward with a long stride and lower the body down and forward.
	v)	The lead leg should be fully flexed with most of the weight on this leg.
	vi)	The rear leg should be slightly flexed — trunk as erect as possible.
Exercise variations		
Free weights	The Squat, Dead Lift, Step Ups with Dumbbells	
Machine systems	Leg Press, Universal Total Hip, Stair Climbing	

Table 6.14: **Gluteus maximus.**

Targeted muscle (prime mover):	Biceps femoris	
Antagonist:	**Quadriceps**	
Palpation:	Lateral posterior side of the femur, near the knee.	
Origin:	Long head — tuberosity of ischium. Short head — central line of femur — linea aspera.	
Insertion:	Head of the fibula and lateral condyle of tibia.	
Muscle action:	Extension of the thigh at the hip. Flexion of the leg at the knee. Outward rotation of the femur.	
Sports action:	Works in association with the other two hamstrings and is used in all running jumping and skipping type movements.	
Kinesiological analysis:	The biceps femoris forms the outer hamstring. Only its long head crosses the hip joint. Its effectiveness as an extensor is in reverse proportion to the degree of flexion of the knee joint. If the knee is sharply flexed, the muscle has insufficient tension to act effectively at the hip joint..	
Muscles that assist the prime mover:		
Semitendinosus	Origin:	Tuberosity of the ischium.
	Insertion:	Upper anterior medial condyle of the tibia.
Semimembranosus	Origin:	Tuberosity of the ischium.
	Insertion:	Posterior surface medial condyle of the tibia.
Gluteus maximus	Origin:	Outer surface of the crest of the ilium, posterior surface of the sacrum and fascia of the lumbar area.
	Insertion:	Gluteal line of femur and iliotibial band of fascia latae.
Common exercise	**The Leg Curl isolates biceps femoris, semitendinosus and semimembranosus.**	
Exercise technique	i)	Lie face down on the bench with the knees just off the end.
	ii)	Adjust the pads to fit the behind the ankles.
	iii)	Bend the knees to curl the pads as high as possible and to the buttocks.
	iv)	Slowly lower, controlling the motion all the way to the start position.
	v)	The hips have a natural tendency to move into hip joint flexion during this exercise.
	vi)	This action raises the origin of the hamstrings, making them more biomechanically effective as knee joint flexors.
Exercise variations:		
Free weights	The Squat High, Block Lunge, Dead lift	
Machine systems	Standing Cable Curl, Hydra Gym Leg Curl (Alt), Leg Press Machine	

Table 6.15: **Biceps femoris.**

Targeted muscle (prime mover):	Rectus femoris	
Antagonist:	**Hamstrings**	
Palpation:	Any place on the anterior surface of the femur.	
Origin:	Anterior-inferior iliac spine of the ilium.	
Insertion:	Top of the patella and patellar ligament to the tibial tuberosity.	
Muscle action:	Flexion of the thigh at the hip. Extension of the leg at the knee.	
Sports action:	The rectus femoris is used in all sports that require hip flexion followed by lower leg extension. It is therefore essential in all explosive movements such as kicking a football, running, jumping etc.	
Kinesiological analysis:	The rectus femoris is the most superficial of the quadriceps group and is the only one of the four that acts at the hip joint.	
Muscles that assist the prime mover:		
Vastus medialis	Origin:	Medial lip of the linea aspera, intertrochanteric line.
	Insertion:	Patella and patellar ligament to the tibial tuberosity.
Vastus lateralis	Origin:	Outer surface of the femur below the greater trochanter and linea aspera of the femur.
	Insertion:	Patella and patellar ligament to the tibial tuberosity.
Vastus intermedius	Origin:	Upper two thirds of the anterior surface of the femur.
	Insertion:	Patella and patellar ligament to the tibial tuberosity.
Common exercise	**The Leg Extension is the most common exercise used for isolating the quadriceps.**	
Exercise technique	i)	Sit on a leg extension machine so the knees are at the end of the bench and let the shins hang vertically.
	ii)	Place the instep of the front of the ankle joint against the rollers.
	iii)	Lean the trunk back to approximately a 45° angle and hold onto the sides of the bench for support.
	iv)	Extend the legs until they are straight but not locked.
	v)	Return to the start position.
Exercise variations:		
Free weights	The Back Squat, The Front Squat, The Lunge	
Machine systems	The Hack Squat, The Close Stance Leg Press, Cable Pulley	

Table 6.16: **Rectus femoris.**

and work intensively on these. Free weights, it is argued, offer better total muscle group conditioning than do machine systems, thereby offering greater economy of training.

Individuality: Some machines are designed to provide variable resistance through the full range of movement. However, to do so they rely on force-angle relationships which are based on estimates from the average person. Individual differences in limb length, point of muscle attachment, muscle architecture, velocity of movement, etc. mean that certain individuals may be restricted in their movements because inappropriate workloads may be applied at various angles. This does not occur with free weights.

Psychological factors: Although not proven, it has been suggested that athletes are more motivated to improve their strength performance using free weights. This is because of the greater satisfaction of improving poundage and personal best performances with loose weights.

Advantages of machine systems

Safety: The loading mechanisms of machine systems are generally enclosed within the structure of the unit. This offers safety advantages that are not present with heavy, loose free weights. This is particularly so with hydraulic loading systems where children may be present.

Some manufacturers also claim that there is less chance of injury through incorrect movements if the range of movements is fixed and the action is guided.

Cheating: As for safety, the fixed movements of many machine systems ensure that correct exercise form is maintained so that cheating cannot occur. This is a particular advantage for beginners and those who tend to take the easy way out.

Compactness: There's little question that most machine systems are more compact and neater than a set of free weights, and are therefore more physically attractive in many gym situations. They also offer more effective use of time because of the ease with which loads and other adjustments can be made. However, the latter claim needs to be seen in perspective, because cost differentials mean that many barbells and dumbbells could be purchased for the price of one machine system unit.

Rehabilitation training: The guided action and variable resistance of some machine systems makes them particularly suited to injury rehabilitation training. Less strain is likely to be put on injured joints than with free weights.

General fitness training: Where specific muscle strength, as in sports-specific training, is not the aim of the program, machine systems may offer more advantage than free weights. Certain systems may be of particular advantage in circuit training.

Variations in Weight Training — Beginner to Advanced

Techniques employed are vital aspects of any weight-training program. Most standard instructional weight training texts have set approaches to both.

Yet just as the amount of load used is increased as an exerciser advances, changes in lifting technique also occur with experience. Some of these variations are not covered in the standard texts. For example:

Feet positioning in the bench press: Commercially made bench-press benches are often only long enough to accommodate the torso to the base of the pelvis in the supine position, leaving the legs to hang over the bench.

The legs can either be positioned flat on the floor, in which case the back is arched, or placed in the air or on the end of the bench, thus flattening the back.

An arched (and unsupported) back is potentially dangerous for the inexperienced or those with lower back problems. Hence, the beginner should be taught either to place the feet on an extension of the bench, or cross the legs in the air with the hips flexed so the back is flattened (Fig. 6.2). On the other hand, an experienced lifter using a heavy weight may need to keep the feet flat on the floor to maintain a wider and more stable base of support.

Use of machines versus free weights:
Machine systems in resistance training have a distinct safety advantage over free weights. The guided action makes it difficult for the beginner to make mistakes. Machine systems also facilitate learning of the correct technique for later progression to free weights. Free weights offer advantages over machine systems in that stabilising and synergistic muscles are used, promoting greater joint strength, stability and co-ordination of movement in the joints used. The preferred progression is therefore from using machine systems to free weights.

Progressions in the squat:
The squat is one of the best overall compound exercises available. But it has inherent dangers, particularly because of the pressure placed on knee ligaments when the knee is flexed beyond 90°. Orthopaedic studies have shown that the shearing force on the knee can increase by up to 7 times that of the weight being carried when the knee is flexed beyond this position.

Other problems with the squat are:
- achieving an effective technique such that the maximum benefits are gained;
- the tendency to cheat in order to carry a heavy load.

For the beginner, any of the standard squat machines can help develop technique. However, the beginner should never be put into the full squat position.

Often, lack of flexibility in the Achilles tendon leads to a tendency to want to place the heels on a raised block. This only exacerbates the problem. Therefore the beginner should be taught to squat only to a point that is comfortable, with the heels on the floor and each patella positioned over the large toe. As flexibility improves and more movement is possible, the squat can, with caution, be taken lower to a depth where position of thighs is parallel to the floor.

Other changes which can be made with advanced training include changes in feet position (toes in, out etc.), changes in the position of the bar (back of neck versus front of chest) and changes in weight used.

Increased sets/decreased reps:
In the early part of a weight-training program, large increases in strength can come from one set of relatively low-resistance exercises. This has the added advantage of minimising muscle soreness and reducing the risk of injury.

As experience is gained, the load should be increased and correct technique maintained. Repetitions can be decreased from 12–15 per set to 6–8 per set and weight increased accordingly. Sets can then be increased as a means of providing greater overload.

Training intensity:
This is the most critical aspect of obtaining results from a weight training program. It is often synonymous with the amount of resistance used — one researcher defines intensity as 'a percentage of momentary ability'. In other words, intensity relates to the degree of muscular fatigue at any given instant. For example, when you start performing a set your momentary ability is high and the intensity or effort is low. Conversely, at the end of the set your momentary ability is low and the intensity is high. The greater the intensity achieved for a given range of repetitions the greater will be the adaptive response from muscle. Unlike cardiovascular training, where different levels of intensity fulfil different requirements, the general rule for weight training is: the harder you train (i.e. the greater the intensity achieved), the greater your results.

The results elicited through weight training are directly related to the degree of muscular fatigue achieved. However, only advanced lifters are capable of, and enjoy, training to exhaustion. For the beginner or the average gym user working to exhaustion isn't appealing. However, for positive changes to occur, the body must at least be stressed beyond intensities to which it is accustomed.

From uniformity to periodisation:
For a beginner, the most important aspect of a weight-training program is learning technique and muscle adaptation. Hence, uniformity of a training program over 2–4 days a week is important, with gradual progressions in resistance, repetitions etc.

For the more advanced exerciser on the other hand, greater advances are made from periodisation; that is, changing the program over a set period of either weeks or months.

A regime of light weights with high repetitions can be used for 3–6 weeks, followed by a period of 3–6 weeks with heavy weights and low repetitions. This can then lead into a third cycle, where the weight is relatively light again, although at a higher level than phase 1. Greater strength developments have been shown using this technique than the uniform training approach.

From 'compound' to 'isolation': Isolation exercises have little value to a beginner exerciser looking for general improvements in muscle tone and health.

With improved general fitness more isolation work may be included in order to improve on specific muscle development. Hence the beginner would concentrate on compound movements, the advanced on a compound/ isolation mix.

Learn lifting technique before progressing to heavy weights: Ensure that the lifter has mastered the technique with lighter weights so that he/she can progress to heavier weights with good form. This will prevent additional muscles being recruited when lifting heavier weights. For example, take the squat, where an inexperienced lifter using too heavy a weight will tend to forward flex the trunk, while at the same time losing some stability at the knee joints, causing them to come together.

For the beginner: Stress caution and avoid exercises involving hyperextension and extreme joint flexion.

Breathe normally throughout the lift: As a general rule, lifters should exhale with the exertion and inhale when lowering the weight. However, there are exceptions to this rule, e.g. an upright row where it does not feel right to breathe out when lifting the weight to the chin and to breathe in when lowering the weight. To overcome these exceptions instructors should encourage participants to keep their mouths open, and to breathe normally throughout the lift.

If a weight trainer does not breathe correctly during a lift, blood pressure can increase dramatically due to what is called a 'valsalva' manoeuvre. This means making an expiratory effort with the glottis closed (the glottis is the space or opening between the vocal cords). Since air cannot escape, intrathoracic pressure increases appreciably, even to the point where it can cause the venae cavae, which return blood to the heart, to collapse. This in turn can cause the person to black out.

Specialist Resistance Training Programs

Traditionally resistance training has been more popular with men wishing to gain strength and muscle hypertrophy. This is no longer the case, as resistance training is now attracting a broad cross section of the general public. Even though the principles remain the same there are idiosyncrancies specific to different target populations with which the instructor should be familiar.

Resistance training for seniors

Strength training programs can help the elderly maintain independence, counter decreases in metabolic rate caused by atrophy of muscle tissue that occurs with ageing, and generally feel better in themselves. The primary emphasis of a program designed for the seniors should be on improving an individual's quality of life — that is, enhancing the ability to carry out normal daily activities with more stamina, strength and energy.

Why should the elderly become involved in strength training? Muscle strength declines, even in trained athletes, after age 60 to 65 years. This decline can lead to immobility, quickened onset of fatigue and a higher incidence of falls and fractures. Statistics show that 40% of people over the age of 65 fall at least once a year and as a result many die from complications arising from fall injuries. Improvements in lower extremity strength can help to reduce this risk. Also, a strong person can rise from a chair in 0.6 seconds, but a weak person may require 6 seconds. For many seniors, simply being able to get out of a chair is of greater importance for quality of life than being able to run across the street.

Arm strength is usually fairly well preserved in the elderly because they use their arm muscles more, even when they are sedentary. Developing leg strength may be more critical because it decreases more rapidly. An emphasis should be placed on the knee and hip extensors because these muscles are used for a multitude of

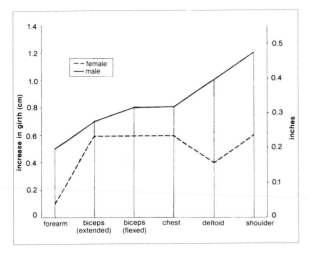

Figure 6.6: **Muscular hypertrophy in females is generally not as great as in males even when the same strength gains have been made.**

activities, and on the dorsiflexors of the foot because these are important for walking. The program should be rounded out with exercises that cover the major muscle groups including the chest, back and trunk muscles.

Because many elderly people have high blood pressure and heart disease concerns, proper breathing is extremely important. If the breath is held, blood pressure may increase and pulse rate may decrease: neither is safe in terms of cardiovascular function. Encourage rhythmic breathing with an emphasis on exhalation during the exertion phase of the lift. Also, avoid any isometric exercises, as these may have adverse cardiovascular effects.

To avoid injury, start with a low weight and work up to heavier weights, reaching a maximum of 80% capacity. The best benefits are seen when elderly exercisers work at 60–80% of maximum capacity. Choose 6–10 exercises encompassing the muscle groups stated above and work 1 to 2 sets of 8–12 repetitions.

Suggested exercises

- Leg Extension
- Cable Hip Extension
- Bench Press
- Seated Military Press
- Abdominal Crunch
- Leg Curl
- Toe Tapping
- Lat Pull Down
- Bicep Curl
- Controlled Back Extension

Weight machines are preferable for the elderly because:

- They eliminate the balance factor — a common problem with the elderly.
- The low back is protected because the user is seated and often belted.
- There are handles to grip (caution against gripping too hard as it can cause elevations in blood pressure).
- Machines are generally weighted lightly, so users can start at a low level.
- The weights increase in small increments.

General guidelines

When encouraging seniors to become involved in resistance exercise, emphasise the improvements in quality of life. Encourage regular workouts — a minimum of two per week with one day of rest in between. Start at a low level and build up slowly; provide supervised weight training sessions, as the elderly will be unfamiliar with the exercises and safety factors involved. Make sure that an adequate active warm-up is performed and that plenty of time is spent stretching at the end, to enhance the flexibility benefit.

Strength training for the elderly can be rewarding for both the client and the instructor, as benefits will be quickly seen and appreciated. How much exercise is too much for this population? A good general guideline is: if people feel more than pleasantly tired the next day after exercise, they are probably doing too much.

Women and resistance training

Women do not have the same capabilities to increase muscular size as men, due to the fact that the average female has ten times less testosterone in her system than the average male. This is paralleled by the fact that female muscle produces less tension per unit volume and has a smaller cross-sectional area in each muscle fibre.

Women have the same potential for strength development as men, although it is through a different mechanism. Females increase their strength by improving the recruitment of motor nerves rather than altering the contractile structures of their muscles.

Some research has shown that when males and females are compared on the basis of strength per unit of lean body mass, females are in fact slightly stronger than men in certain areas such as the hips and legs. However, until recently women have shied away from weight training because of their fear of developing large bulging muscles.

Women can weight train without fear of large increases in muscle size. Research on muscle size difference with training between men and women is shown in Figure. 6.5.

In a study involving a group of untrained college men and women, the subjects were given a 10-week weight training program. Before training, the women's strength was around 25–28% lower than that of the men, although when body weight was taken into consideration, there were no gender differences in strength. After training, strength improved significantly (i.e. 5–25%) and equally in both groups. Yet while muscle size increased significantly in the men, there was no significant increase in size for women.

Prepubescent strength training

The National Strength and Conditioning Association's (NSCA) position paper on prepubescent strength training has prepared guidelines that state that strength training may begin at any age. It states that commencement age is dependent on the child undergoing a physical examination and on him/her having the emotional maturity to take direction from the trainer. Further research is required, but at present the use of higher repetitions and sets with lower loads is most appropriate. The NSCA recommends 6–15 repetitions per set and 1RM testing should never be attempted at this age.

A model training session for prepubescent children would be performed 3 times per week. Each session should consist of a warm-up, 30 min. weight exercises, 20 min. run, 20 min. team game, then a cool-down. The session should stress total body development and should include exercises using the child's own bodyweight such as dips and chins.

Guidelines for Weight Training

The following are some guidelines for the administration of weight training programs:

🏃 At least 5 minutes of warm-up (see Chapter 4) should be carried out before lifting weights. This includes stretching and loosening-up exercises of gradually increasing intensity.

🏃 Particular attention should be paid to safety and to correct exercise procedure. Individual counselling is advisable to assess structural weakness or abnormalities in participants.

🏃 Weight standards should be determined at the outset for each participant; these should then be adjusted according to improvement.

🏃 A strength training routine should involve the use of the overload principle, i.e. progressively heavier weights or an increasing number of repetitions and/or sets.

🏃 Strength training should not be confused with aerobic conditioning and no suggestion should be made that strength training or body building alone will significantly improve aerobic fitness.

🏃 Heavy resistance should not be used until proper lifting techniques are perfected.

🏃 Individual record cards should be available for participants so that workouts can be standardised and efforts recorded. Regular monitoring of cards by an instructor and regular consultations with the client should be carried out.

Movement Mechanics

Incorporating Potentially Dangerous Exercises, Back Care, Injury Recognition and Prevention

Fitness leaders must have a clear understanding of the basic mechanics of the musculoskeletal system in order to assess which exercises may be considered potentially dangerous. This knowledge is critical in the selection of safer exercise alternatives. Movement mechanics are also of vital importance in understanding the back and dealing with the common problem of back pain. Finally, in order to recognise and prevent exercise-related injury, a thorough knowledge of common injuries and their causes is vital.

The Mechanics of Joint and Muscle Action

In any mechanism the components are continuously placed under stress, some more than others. If this stress becomes too great through over-use or excess loading, weaknesses are likely to develop. An analogy is in driving a motor car: if a car is only driven on short trips at a moderate pace, minor structural weaknesses can be masked. But if it is taken on a long drive at varying speeds, minor defects are likely to show up. So it is with the body. At mild exercise levels, small structural defects such as differences in leg length (which are surprisingly common) are unlikely to be noticed. But if the exerciser takes up a substantial endurance training program for example, chronic injury is more likely to result.

Even for the structurally sound, some exercises can place excessive strain on muscles and joints. If this happens, wear and tear can result, degenerative changes may set in and damage can result. Consequently, the need for understanding the mechanics of movement arises.

Human motion is made possible through intricate interactions between the muscular and skeletal systems, whereby contracting muscles pull on bones that are arranged in a series of simple mechanical lever systems or links (see Chapter 1), collectively referred to as the kinetic link system. Lever systems are employed to effectively shift a given load through a given distance and the

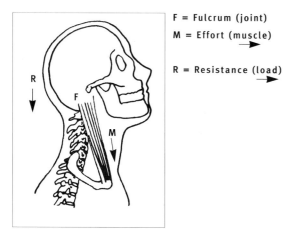

F = Fulcrum (joint)

M = Effort (muscle)

R = Resistance (load)

Figure 7.1: **First class lever.**

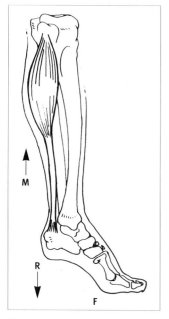

Figure 7.2: **Second class lever.**

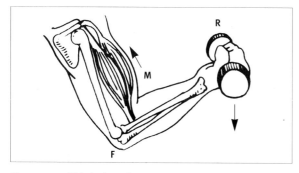

Figure 7.3: **Third class lever.**

type of lever system employed determines the function of a joint. All lever systems have a fulcrum (the joint), a rigid lever arm (the bone) and a point for the application of the force needed to move the lever arm (the insertion point of the muscle).

The position of the joint (the fulcrum) in relation to the point of muscle insertion and the lever arm determines the type of lever system being used.

There are three main types of levers in the body. Some are designed for stability and lifting heavy loads, ie. first and second class levers, whereas third class levers are designed to generate high rotational speed.

First class lever

The fulcrum (joint) always lies between the effort (muscle) and the resistance (load). This is the most efficient form of lever for moving heavy loads (Fig. 7.1), an example being the movement of the head where the skull pivots on the Atlas (1st cervical vertebra).

Second class lever

In this instance the resistance (R) always lies between the fulcrum (F) and the muscle (M) (Fig. 7.2). An example would be pushing or lifting a wheelbarrow or lifting the body weight up onto the toes by plantar flexion of the feet.

Third class lever

Here the muscular effort is applied between the resistance and the fulcrum providing the least efficient mechanical advantage (Fig. 7.3). Most of the joints involved in locomotion of the body are third class levers. This type of joint is designed to generate angular speed where a small amount of movement at the fulcrum results in much greater movement at the distal end of the lever arm. An example is the contraction of the biceps to lift the hand.

If excessive strain (force or weight) is applied to the lever in any of these three systems, the force placed on the fulcrum is increased, resulting in wear and tear on the joint. Hence the aim of an exercise program should be to optimise the relationship between muscle strength and joint integrity.

Potentially Dangerous Exercises

Aerobics and fitness training is a rapidly changing field. Only in the last five to ten years have exercise scientists looked closely at the benefits and concerns of relatively new exercise forms such as exercise to music classes. As the fitness industry continues to grow, and more unfit, overweight, sedentary individuals take on structured exercise programs, it is even more important to identify which exercises tend to cause injury. To ensure that exercise programs and floor classes are effective and safe, fitness instructors must be up-to-date not only on potentially dangerous exercises, but why the danger exists and how to modify exercises for safer alternatives.

Understanding the danger

Consistency in an industry adds credibility. If all fitness instructors have a sound understanding of what constitutes an exercise danger, programs will become safer and participants will not be asking 'Why does one instructor often do that exercise and now I am told it's dangerous?'

The first step to providing safer exercise programs is a willingness to change in accordance with current information. Just because an instructor has been doing an exercise for a long time doesn't mean the exercise is safe. Instructors should keep in mind that there are no lists which contain every potentially dangerous exercise. Instructors must try to understand the elements which increase risk and the areas where injuries are most likely to occur. Then, each instructor can evaluate their own exercises and determine which ones need to be modified.

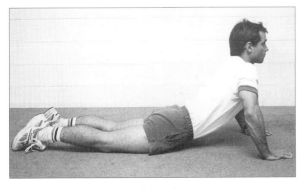

Figure 7.4: **Cobra stretch (above) — extreme hyperextension.**

There are conflicting opinions, even among the 'experts' about which exercises are dangerous. If an instructor has a clear understanding of why a movement may be dangerous, he/she can then listen to conflicting opinions and make an educated decision.

Exercise safety is a priority in all programs, therefore fitness instructors should keep in mind three primary factors:

1. The participants: Every individual is different in terms of strength, flexibility, skill, coordination, weight, fitness level and speed of learning. Some may be more prone to injury because of anatomical, structural or other physiological factors. Often these factors may be present without the individual (and hence the instructor) being aware of them.

Also, wearing inappropriate shoes or no shoes at all is a potential danger, and a leading cause of lower leg pain and injury. Avoid letting people exercise bare-footed, and encourage the wearing of proper, well-designed shoes. There is no such thing as the perfect shoe that is suitable for everyone; wherever possible professional advice should be sought. Two basic characteristics of a good shoe are a comfortable overall fit and good structural stability that is specific for a given activity.

2. The instructor: The instructor can control the degree of safety of an exercise: for example, speed of movement, number of repetitions, sequencing of exercises, cueing of changes, and the amount of impact. The instructor who is up-to-date understands these variables and uses them effectively when planning exercise programs.

3. The goal: The primary goal of an exercise program is to improve an individual's overall wellbeing. This can include improvements in both health and sports-related physical fitness, as well as psychological aspects like self-esteem and sense of accomplishment. In general, life-long fitness should be encouraged; this is best achieved through gradual and sustainable program increments that are considered safe and effective. Finishing an exercise program with a sore back, sore knees, uncomfortable shins, or feeling exhausted does not encourage program adherence. Overload is a basic exercise principle, but there is a difference between

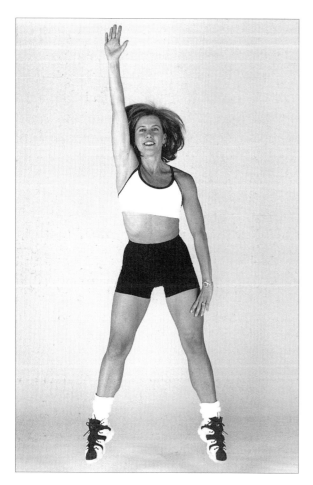

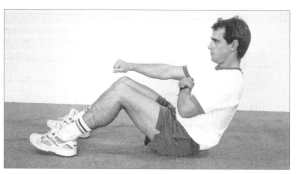

Figure 7.6: **V sits or free back are not recommended.**

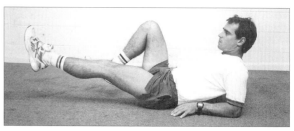

Figure 7.7: **Bicycling — a hip flexor exercise more than an abdominal exercise.**

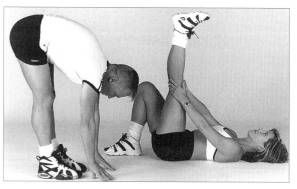

Figure 7.8: **Toe touching to stretch the hamstrings — a safer alternative is executed lying supine.**

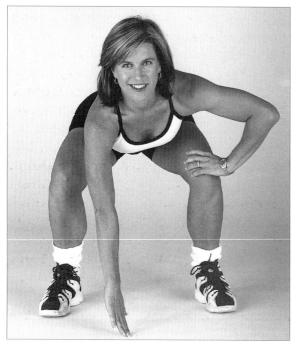

Figure 7.5: **Power jump** (top). **On landing, excessive load can be placed on the knees** (above).

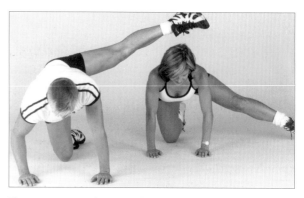

Figure 7.9: **Long lever and the safer short lever alternative.**

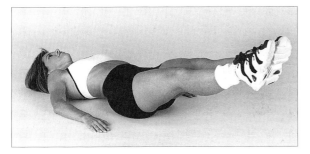

Figure 7.10: **Long lever exercises that place stress on the lower back.**

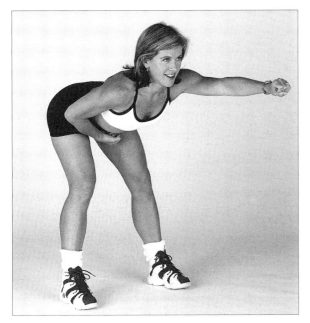

Figure 7.11: **Long lever exercises that place stress on the lower back.**

damaging pain and overload. Although achieving sufficient overload may be accompanied by slight discomfort, it should not be painful.

Movement evaluation

Elements that commonly cause injury are explained below:

Extreme movements: These are movements that go beyond a safe range of motion, either in distance or direction. Most movements which involve hyperflexion and hyperextension are considered extreme and potentially dangerous, especially when loaded. For example, the 'cobra stretch' (lying face down, hands under the shoulders and fully extending the arms, pushing up to

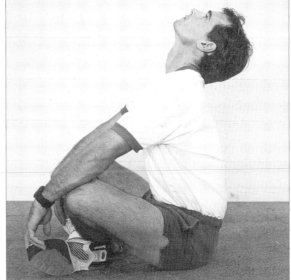

Figure 7.12: **Neck hyperextension places excessive stress on the cervical vertebrae.**

bend the back) places the lower back in an extreme extended position (Fig. 7.4). The uncontrolled use of momentum during exercise may also lead to extreme ranges of motion at the moving joint — this is referred to as ballistic movement.

Ballistic movements are movements performed rapidly, without control, going beyond the normal range of motion. Often an exercise may be safe, but when performed rapidly it becomes unsafe, especially when a long lever arm is involved. For example, rapidly swinging the arms to mobilise the shoulders places stress on the connective tissue in the shoulder joint and does not promote mobility or flexibility.

Excessive loading: Movements may involve excessive load to a joint or muscle group. For example, during a floor class, 'power jumps' — jumping up and touching the floor with the hands. On landing, an excessive load is applied to the knees if they are forced to bend beyond a safe (90°) angle (Fig. 7.5). Excessive loading through resistance training is also a common cause of injury.

Sustained movements: Any movement or position that involves sustained stress on a muscle group or joint. For example, sitting in a V-sit position with feet on the floor and the back unsupported (free back) to

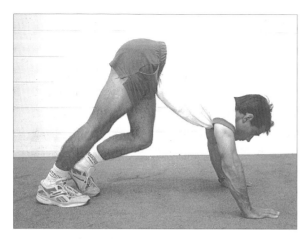

Figure 7.13: (above) Sprint Start — problems with dizziness, blood pressure and shoulders.

work the abdominal muscles (Fig. 7.6). In this position, there is excessive, sustained load on the lower back from the heavy upper body lever, causing high intervertebral pressure. The result — lower back pain.

Repetitive movements: Excessive repetitions (even of safe exercises) can cause pain, discomfort and injury. During floor work in an exercise class, change exercise frequently before pain is felt. During upright cardiovascular work, use no more than 32 consecutive footstrike patterns and no more than 8 consecutive foot-strikes on one leg.

Imbalance: Working one muscle group excessively without working the opposing muscle group.

Wrong selection: Exercises where the targeted muscle is not responsible for the primary movement. For example, the iliopsoas muscle (hip flexor) is responsible for hip flexion, not the rectus abdominis. As such, the bicycling motion shown in Figure 7.7, which is often

thought to strengthen the lower abdominals, primarily strengthens the hip flexors.

A second example is the lack of tibialis anterior strengthening and stretching to balance the calf work often done in aerobic classes. This can cause a muscular imbalance that may lead to pain in the lower leg.

Principles of movement

In addition to the elements that increase risk, there are several principles of movement (and physics!) which must be understood:

The force of gravity: Gravitational forces are used advantageously in some exercise protocols like plyometrics; however, inappropriate application of these forces can increase injury risk significantly. Because of gravity, the force applied to a joint can be increased and become excessive. For example, standing in a forward flexed position to stretch the hamstrings causes a substantial rise in disc pressure and increases the strain on back extensor muscles and ligaments. A much safer hamstring stretch can be achieved lying on the back (see Fig. 7.8).

Gravity, with respect to non-equipment exercises, can work in our favour by providing a small amount of 'built in resistance'. For example, abdominal crunches involve lifting the upper body against the force of gravity, hence increasing the effectiveness of the exercise.

Lever lengths and joint stress: The long levers of the body, i.e. straight legs and arms, operate as third class levers with the hip and shoulder as fulcrums. The longer the third class lever arm, the greater is the muscular force required for movement, hence the longer the lever arm the greater the stress placed on a joint. For example, a gluteal exercise with a straight leg out to the

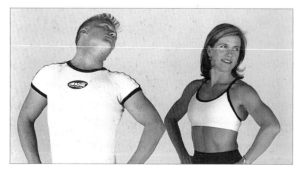

Figure 7.14: **Momentum.**

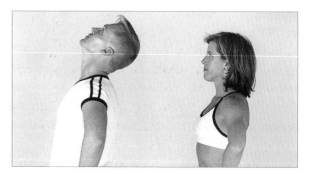

Figure 7.15: **Hyperextension.**

side is a long lever movement, which places excess stress on the lower back (see Fig. 7.9). Figures 7.10 and 7.11 show additional long lever positions that place high stress on the lower back. Combining short and long lever movements and shortening the lever when joint stress is suspected will make your workouts safer.

The final step in evaluation

Each of the elements and movement principles above are related to the risk of an exercise. The final step in the risk evaluation process is to consider the effectiveness of the movement. Ask yourself why you are doing the exercise — aerobic conditioning, muscular strength, strength endurance, flexibility, mobility? Then determine what muscle group you are trying to work. Does the exercise accomplish these things?

Your aim is to develop highly effective programs that are low risk. Each exercise in your program should aim to meet these criteria. Aerobic exercises should be strenuous enough for people to achieve their target heart rates, but not so strenuous that they are working at a fatigue level that risks injury or discomfort. Floor exercises should be done in a slow, controlled manner, work through a full range of motion, provide sufficient overload within a short period of time, and with limited repetitions and frequent changes of position.

Modifying PDEs: The final step in providing safe and effective exercise programs is being able to modify or replace potentially dangerous exercises (PDEs) with a safe alternative.

Learning about PDEs can be frustrating at first, when you discover that half the exercises you've been doing for years are potentially dangerous. However, don't become disillusioned — you may have to modify a position or change an exercise altogether, but keep in mind that for every exercise you sacrifice in the name of safety there is an alternative. Go back to the question you asked yourself, 'Why am I doing this exercise?' If it was for abdominal toning, what are some other ways you can achieve that goal with less risk? Sometimes making the program (e.g. an aerobic class) safer is simply a matter of slowing down the pace! Slower, controlled movements working the full range of motion will always be safer and more effective than rapid ones in both aerobic work and muscle conditioning. Besides, what's the hurry? A good

workout should be just that — a workout not a wipeout.

Use the following 'Safer Moves' segment as a guideline for areas in which potentially dangerous exercises occur. Remember, there are so many exercises, variations and combinations that no list will ever include all the dangerous exercises. It is up to the instructor to understand, evaluate and modify!

Safer Moves

Please note: The male model in the illustrations on pages 87–96 is doing the dangerous exercise, the female model is doing a modified safer version.

Head and neck

Momentum: Avoid rapid or jerking movements (Fig. 7.14). Instead, use controlled movement from side to side or up and down.

Hyperextension: Neck rolls or stretches in a backward direction should be avoided, due to stress on the cervical vertebrae (Fig. 7.15). Also, beware when doing exercises on all fours because there is a tendency to hyperextend the neck to see the instructor (Fig. 7.16). Turn side-on, maintaining a neutral head position and rotating it slightly to observe the instructor.

Loaded or extreme flexion: This also causes excessive stress on the cervical vertebrae. Replace the 'plough' with the cat stretch (Fig. 7.17). Avoid standing on the shoulders at all times (Fig. 7.18) and encourage participants not to pull the head when supporting it during abdominal work. Avoid pulling the head to stretch the back of the neck.

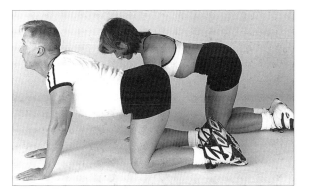

Figure 7.16: **Hyperextension.**

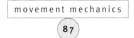

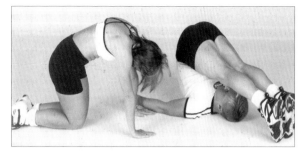

Figure 7.17: **Loaded or extreme flexion.**

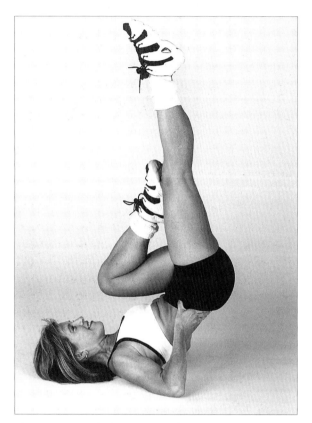

Figure 7.18: **Loaded or extreme flexion.**

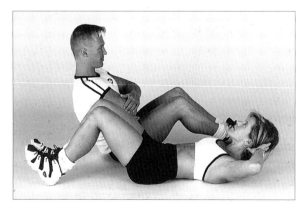

Figure 7.19: **Loaded or extreme flexion.**

Shoulders

Sustained, repetitive shoulder isolations: Small movements with the arms out to the side are examples of repeated shoulder isolations (Fig. 7.20). Work full range of motion, varying between short and long levers.

Momentum: Rapid swinging of outstretched arms places undue stress on the shoulder joints (Fig. 7.21). Work within the normal range of motion and try to avoid any rapid swinging or pulling movements, especially with the arms outstretched.

Impingement: Excessive, repetitive (normally more than fifty) arm movements in the same direction, particularly overhead or to the front or side can cause impingement in the shoulder area. Limit the number of repetitions and change arm positions frequently. In addition, keep the arms slightly forward rather than straight overhead during upward movements.

Trunk/torso

Free back: Supporting the weight of the upper torso in positions such as that shown in Figure 7.22a. can cause high intervertebral pressure and stress on the lower back. In addition, to effectively work the abdominal muscles, they should generally be worked through a full range of motion, rather than sustaining an isometric contraction. The danger is further increased when a twisting motion is added (Fig. 7.22b.) or when the feet are off the ground as in the 'jackknife' position (Fig. 7.22c.).

Double straight leg raises: Supporting the long lever of the legs in this position (Fig.7.23a.) causes stress on the lower back and can lead to back pain. Also avoid variations of this position such as scissors and flutter kicks (Fig. 7.23b.). Because the prime movers for these movements are the hip flexors, the abdominal muscles receive little benefit from these exercises.

Twisting on a fixed base: These movements apply excessive rotational torque to the lower back. When standing and twisting (Fig. 7.24a.), one heel should be raised. Rapid and/or repetitive twisting should not be performed when seated (Fig. 7.24b.). It is more effective to perform slow, controlled twisting movements with the back safely supported on the floor.

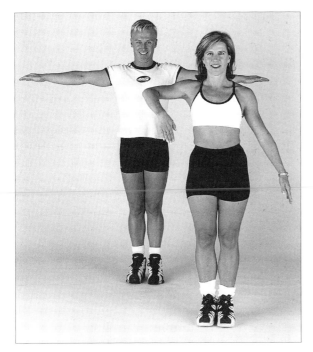

Figure 7.20: **Sustained repetitive isolations.**

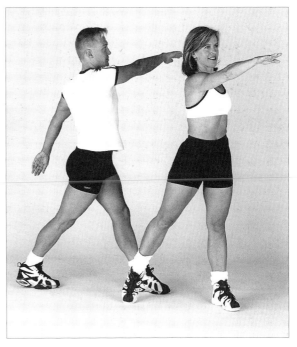

Figure 7.21: **Momentum.**

Forward flexion with and without rotation: Forward flexion (Fig.7.25a.) increases pressure on the discs and ligaments of the lower back by more than three times body weight. Rotation with forward flexion (Fig.7.25b.) further increases torque and pressure. Triceps and rhomboid exercises should be done more upright (Fig.7.25c.). Clapping under the thigh can encourage forward flexion (Fig.7.25e.) so a straight back position should be encouraged, or modify the exercise by clapping on top of the thigh. When seated to stretch the adductor or hamstring muscles (Fig. 7.25d.), the back should remain straight, not rounded. If stretching the back, controlled rounding should be done with knees bent or crossed.

Sprint start position: Commonly used to stretch the calves and for aerobic work. This position has at least three potential dangers: 1) the neck is hyperextended to see the instructor; 2) if lowered, the head falls below the level of the heart causing a blood rush to the head; and 3) there is a sustained isometric contraction of the arms to support the body, causing both discomfort and increased chest pressure which can result in cardiovascular irregularities. Stretch the calves in a seated or standing position (Fig. 7.26a.) and do the aerobic work upright (Fig. 7.26b.) — it is as effective but safer!

Hyperextension: While some back hyperextension work is necessary to strengthen the back muscles and stretch the opposing muscle groups, pain can result if the position is extreme.

When extending the back in a prone position go no further than resting on the elbows (Fig. 7.27). Avoid lifting both upper and lower body off the ground simultaneously — alternate instead (Fig. 7.28). Keep the back on the ground during pelvic tilts (Fig. 7.29). Avoid sagging the abdominal area when working on all fours or performing pushups (Fig. 7.30). Be careful not to hyperextend in exercises while performing calf stretches or during shoulder work (Figs. 7.31 and 7.32).

Excessive lateral flexion: Bending too far to the side without support (standing or seated — Fig. 7.33a. and b. places stress on the lower back from a lateral angle. Always use the arm for support.

Knee

Deep knee bends and other positions of extreme knee flexion: High stresses are placed on the knee joint if it is bent beyond 90°. Deep squats (Fig.7.35a.), power jumps where the end position is touching the floor (Fig.7.35b.), hip flexor stretches with hands on the floor (Fig.7.36a.), stepping into a lunge (Fig.7.36b.),

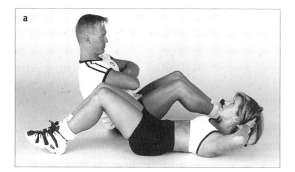

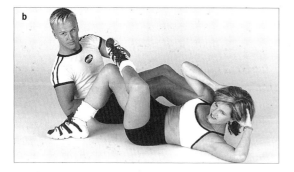

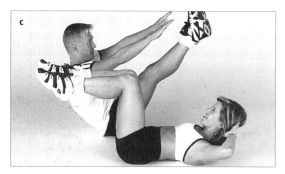

Figure 7.22: Free back.

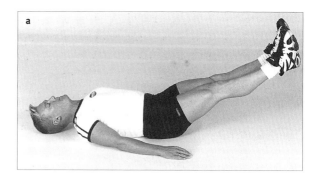

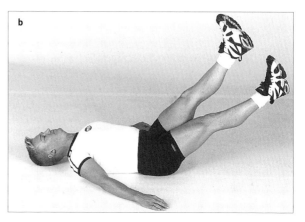

Figure 7.23: Double leg raise.

and adductor stretching where the knee is excessively bent (Fig.7.36c.), can all potentially cause damage.

When the knee is flexed beyond 90^0, the force on the joint can increase by up to 7 times body weight. This compression on the knee joint is exaggerated further if a weight is being lifted while in such a position. Pressure is put on part of the kneecap (patella) which is not well nourished. The result can be excessive wearing, and a 'click' as the joint surfaces slide past each other. Ultimately, there'll be knee pain.

On the other hand, the squat is one of the few exercises which incorporates the large muscles of the thighs in both heavy eccentric and concentric contractions. For this reason it resembles real-life and sports actions more, probably, than any other quadriceps exercise.

Changing one's stance from narrow to wide, toes in to toes out, and shifting weight from high on the shoulders to low on the shoulders or in front of the body, can vary the effort on the legs and back.

Taking everything into consideration, the conclusions of a National Strength and Conditioning Association forum on squatting are:

- If carried out correctly, the squat is one of the best compound exercises there is.
- The dangers of the full squat are in the execution of the exercise. Dangerous techniques include:
  - bouncing out of the bottom fully flexed position;
  - moving too quickly in the descent phase;
  - not keeping the centre of gravity over the middle of the feet;
  - carrying too much weight;
  - bending too far foward during the movement;
  - relaxing at the bottom of the squat before starting to stand up again.
- Although the full squat is probably not dangerous for the experienced when carried out correctly, there is little benefit in the beginner venturing any deeper than the position of legs-parallel-to-the-floor.

- The depth of the squat should be determined by the purpose of the exercise. Quarter squats, for example, recruit muscles as in jogging. The parallel squat recruits muscles used in sprinting and cycling.

- There may be some danger in adolescents squatting during a growth spurt (most likely 14–16 years) because of ligament 'looseness' which occurs at this age.

- While squatting to a bench may help define a safe range for the action, it could cause problems because of:
  - jarring of the spine and coccyx;
  - the tendency to relax, then bounce out of the bottom position;
  - a shift in body weight from bench to the beginning of the upward movement, causing strain.

The NSCA group also agreed on a number of points of technique in squatting with weights:

- Face the squat rack when using weights rather than back in, so that the rack can be seen more safely after squatting.

- Place feet shoulder-width apart or more.

- Avoid excessive upper torso lean. Keep hips directly under the bar, head up.

- Control the rate of descent to approximately 30⁰ per second.

- Use 3 'spotters' if squatting with a heavy weight (one each side and one behind).

- Keep feet flat on the floor (don't use a board under the feet). If flexibility isn't up to the job, develop it by gradually extending the depth of the squat.

- Don't 'bounce' out of the bottom position; instead, accelerate out of it in order to use the quadriceps as much as possible.

- Prevent the knees moving forward excessively during the action (they should be above the centre of the feet).

- Individuals with weak backs, potential or confirmed, should use belts and ensure good form.

- Avoid exhausting the abdominals and lower back before squatting as this can weaken the movement and lead to possible injury.

Incorrect knee alignment: The hurdler's stretch (Fig.7.37a.), poor technique in side to side movement (Fig.7.37b.), rapid directional changes and knee circling (Fig.7.37c.) may all cause a twisting of the knee which can lead to injury. Slow down directional changes, align the centre of the knee directly over the middle of the foot when bending and make sure rotation comes from the hip, not the knee.

Excessive knee extension: Avoid hyperextending or locking the knee during movements such as that shown in (Fig.7.38a.) also be aware of this during other activities like cycling and rowing. Leaning on the knee of a straight leg (Fig.7.38b.) can cause excessive knee extension and is potentially dangerous. Keep the knees soft and do not emphasise placing the heel on the floor when stepping backwards.

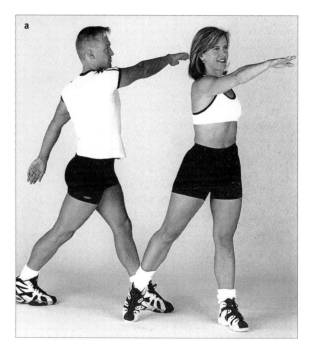

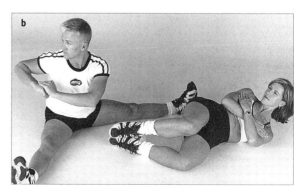

Figure 7.24: **Twisting on a fixed base.**

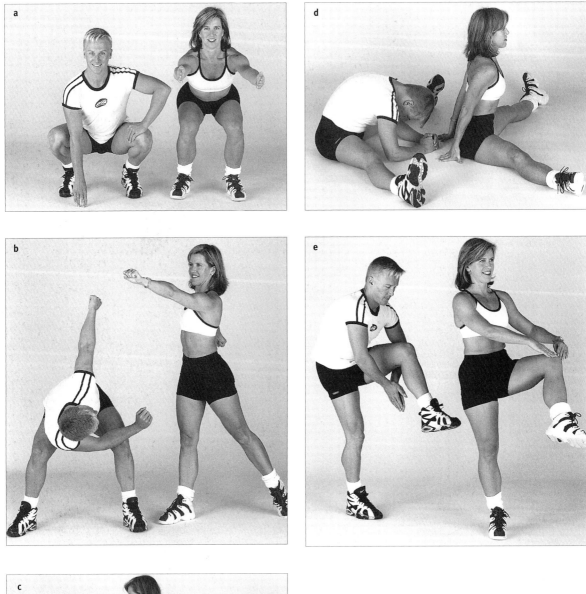

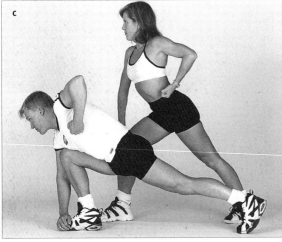

Figure 7.25(a–e): **Forward flexion with and without**

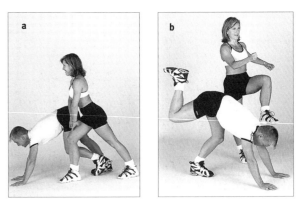

Figure 7.26 (a–b): **Sprint start position.**

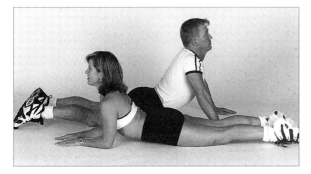

Figure 7.27: Hyperextension.

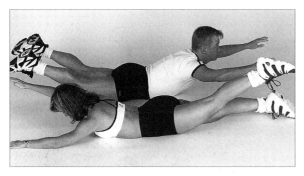

Figure 7.28: Hyperextension.

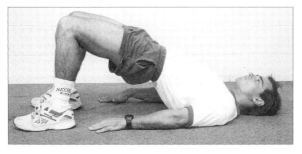

Figure 7.29: Hyperextension.

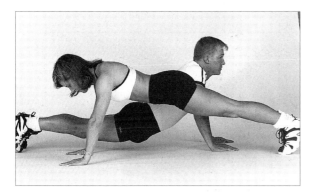

Figure 7.30: Hyperextension.

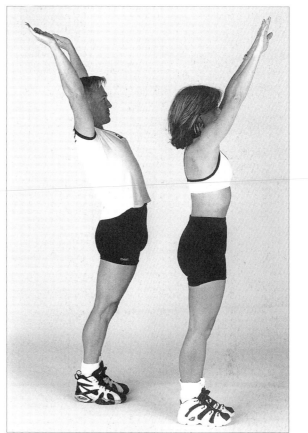

Figure 7.31: Hyperextension.

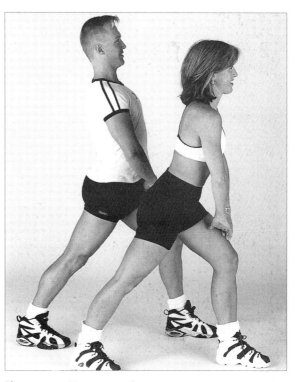

Figure 7.32: Hyperextension.

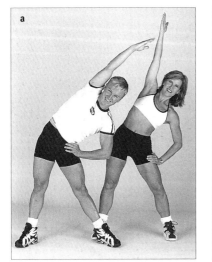
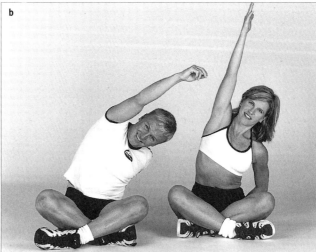

Figure 7.33: **Excessive lateral flexion.**

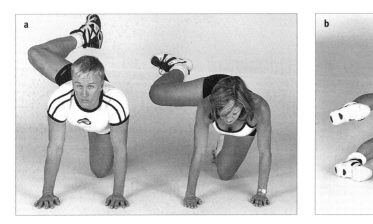

Figure 7.34: **Abduction at 90° angle.**

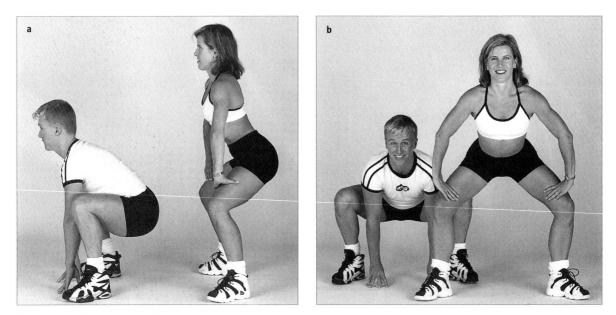

Figure 7.35: **Extreme knee flexion.**

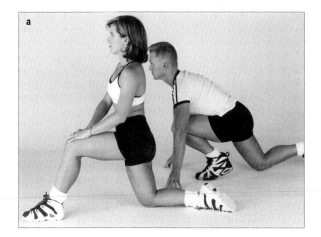

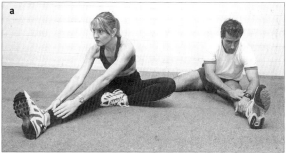

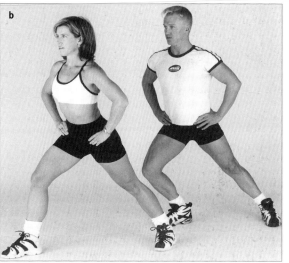

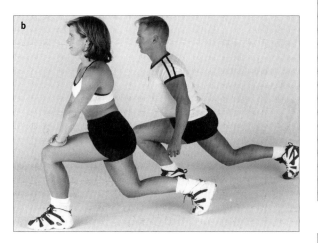

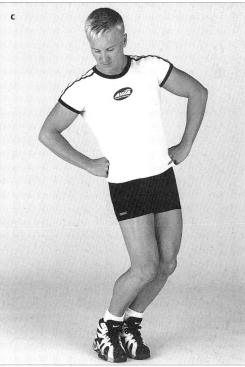

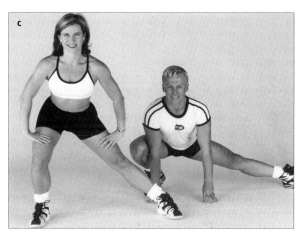

Figure 7.36: **Extreme knee flexion**

Figure 7.37: **Incorrect knee alignment.**

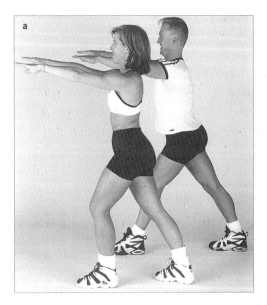

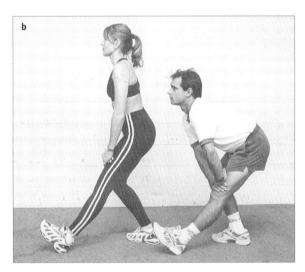

Figure 7.38: **Excessive knee extension.**

Lower leg/ankle/foot

Repetitive stress: Lower leg pain and injuries to the ankle and foot are often the result of an excessive number of repetitions of the same foot strike pattern.

🏃 Do no more than 32 consecutive footstrike patterns at one time.

🏃 Do no more than 8 consecutive footstrike patterns on one leg (that is, no more than 4 hops or jumps on one leg) at a time.

Do not do full tracks with one foot-strike pattern (i.e. jogging on the spot) with only arm variations. Frequent foot pattern changes are most important to reduce repetitive impact stress.

The sit-up or the crunch — which is the better?

The abdominal area seems to attract controversial exercises. Many types of exercises that involve the abdominal muscles are available to the Fitness Leader including the old-fashioned straight leg sit-up, the bent knee full sit-up, full sit-ups with the feet anchored, straight leg raises and an assortment of straight leg raises with scissor and flutter kicking. All of these exercises contain one or more elements of risk.

There is an abundance of research that shows strengthening the abdominal muscles can help prevent low back pain. However, some exercises can have adverse effects; selecting the correct type of abdominal exercise is therefore, an important factor.

In relation to the straight leg sit-up, research clearly shows that:

• when the legs are straight, the hip flexor muscles, and not the abdominal muscles, act as the prime movers in the exercise;
• anterior diplacement of the fifth lumbar vertebra over the sacrum during the exercise can cause disc pressure problems.

The bent knee full sit-up was proposed to get around this by putting the psoas and other hip flexors 'on the slack' thus reducing the adverse effects of their contraction. However, electromyographical (EMG) studies have shown that the psoas is active in parts of the bent knee sit-up and this could shorten and tighten the hip flexors more because it involves them in a shorter range of motion. A further problem with the full bent knee sit-up is the amount of intra-disc pressure found around the third lumbar disc. This pressure was found to be equal to that in forward flexion movements that are also contraindicated. Doing full sit-ups with the feet anchored again primarily involves the hip flexors, meaning that the abdominal muscles are probably used to no more than 30% of their efficiency.

Research determined that one of the most efficient exercises for training the abdominal muscles is 'The Crunch'. The crunch, where the trunk is flexed no more than 30^0, is a safe and effective exercise that does not place undue strain on the back area.

The Crunch: It has been shown that in either the bent leg or straight leg version of the sit-up, the abdominal muscles are essentially only used in the first third of the movement. So doing a full sit-up in either case is not warranted if abdominal strength is the objective.

A 'crunch', where the trunk is flexed no more than 30°, is a better choice of exercise than a full sit-up (see the female in Fig.7.22 a, b, c.). These crunch exercises have been shown to recruit as many abdominal motor units as the full sit-up, but lack the potential disc pressure problems.

How useful is the inclined sit-up board? Little research has been done on the effectiveness of the sit-up board for working abdominal muscles. Work that has been done shows these boards may be no more effective for the abdominal muscles than working on a level surface. This is because trunk flexion with legs anchored primarily involves the hip flexor muscles, meaning that abdominals are probably used to no more than about 30% of their efficiency. Using a sit-up board with feet anchored is thought to have a similar effect.

Some manufacturers have attempted to overcome this by having boards where knees are bent over a knee rest. This causes other muscles (calves, hamstrings) to be involved in gripping the legs and produces an effect similar to holding the feet down. An ordinary sit-up action from the floor with hips flexed and feet tucked under the buttocks still seems to offer the best of all worlds.

Back extension exercises

There are some 48 muscles in the region of the lower back alone, many of which are used infrequently. Sudden stress on these muscles can lead to problems, hence all exercises should be performed correctly. Hyperextension of the lower back while lying prone with both arms and legs raised simultaneously should be avoided.

A progression of safe exercises for strengthening the lower back while minimising strain is outlined below. They are performed whilst in the prone position (face down):

1. Lock the heels and buttocks together and hold 5–10 seconds, then relax. This tones some of the lower back muscles without placing any strain on the vertebral joints.
2. Progress to alternate leg lifts, which strengthen the hamstrings and lower back.
3. To strengthen the muscles of the cervical and thoracic spine, place the hands behind the head and lift the head and shoulders. Cross the legs to prevent lifting them.
4. A progression of the above is to lift the shoulders and place the hands behind the back.
5. Progress to modified push-ups by raising only the head and shoulders and keeping the hips on the floor. (Caution: this should not be carried out by anyone with an excessive lordosis or 'sway back'.)
6. As an advanced exercise, place the hips over a pillow or bench and lift the legs alternately to a horizontal position.

Back Pain

Statistics show that 8 out of 10 people will suffer some form of back pain at some stage of their lives, the most common area being the lower back, or lumbosacral spine. There are four areas to work on to overcome or avoid developing back pain: posture and daily movement habits, strengthening the abdominals, strengthening the back, and stretching the back. Before discussing each of these, it is important to review the anatomy of the back.

Posture and daily movement habits

It is hardly surprising that we suffer so much back pain — our backs are affected by how we sit, stand, bend and lift.

Typically, people stand with their shoulders slouched forward, one leg bent (taking the majority of body weight on the straight leg), and with an exaggerated lumbar curvature. This can precipitate back pain. We should try to stand more upright, allowing our spine to have its natural curvature. Shoulders should be slightly back and both feet should be evenly on the ground. With this corrected posture, you can stand comfortably for longer periods of time without aggravating your back.

Bending and lifting incorrectly can also cause back pain. Bending from the waist to vacuum, garden, lift, or pick something up can cause or aggravate back problems.

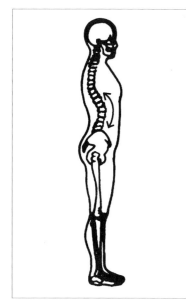

Figure 7.39a: **Lordosis.**

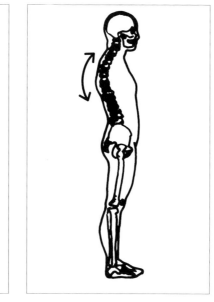

Figure 7.39b: **Kyphosis.**

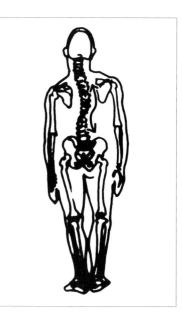

Figure 7.39c: **Scoliosis.**

Try to ensure that the equipment you are using (vacuum cleaner, rake, shovel, etc.) allows you to stand as upright as possible. When lifting, it is important to have the load as close to the body as possible before starting to lift. Bending and lifting should always involve the knees. This allows the strong quadricep and hamstring muscles of the thighs to do the work, rather than the erector spinae.

Anatomy of the back

The spinal column consists of 24 movable bones and 7 less flexible ones (Fig.7.40). These are categorised into five regions as follows:

1. Cervical: consisting of the first 7 vertebrae.
2. Thoracic: includes 12 vertebrae, from the first to last pair of ribs.
3. Lumbar: consists of the 5 largest vertebrae of the-spinal column.
4. Sacral: links the spine to the pelvis. The sacrum is a wedge-shaped bone consisting of 5–7 fused verte-brae.
5. Coccygeal: consists of 2–4 fused vertebrae often referred to as the tail bone.

The vertebral column is like a string of beads that are separated by a thick fibrous structure called the inter-vertebral disc. These discs are pliable; they act as shock absorbers while also allowing for flexibility and move-ment of the spine in different directions.

The vertebral column is held together by strong lig-aments and supported by muscles. With inactivity and age, the discs and ligaments may harden, leading to poor flexibility and eventually back pain.

Other reasons for back pain include:

*   weak abdominal muscles due to a sedentary lifestyle and subsequent poor posture;
*   weak back extensors, which again are due to lack of exercise and poor posture;
*   tightening of the hamstring muscles from excessive running training in the absence of specific flexibil-ity work;
*   biomechanical factors such as leg length differ-ences.

Abnormal spinal postures

The spine should have a normal 'S' curvature when viewed laterally; it should be straight up and down when viewed from a posterior aspect in the sagittal plane. There are three abnormal variations:

1. Lordosis: Excessive curvature in the lumbar spine when viewed laterally. Can be caused by tight hip flex-ors pulling down on the anterior (front) side of the pelvis and tight lumbar extensors pulling up on the pos-terior side of the pelvis. Common in gymnasts, ballet dancers, pregnant women, and abdominally obese men (see Fig. 7.39a).

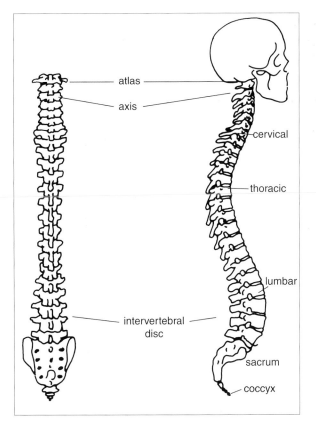

Figure 7.40: **Vertebrae and vertebral column.**

left sides of the body, limb length differences, or heredity. Strengthening and stretching of the affected muscle groups and considering orthotics in the case of limb length differences may correct the problem. Early diagnosis improves chances of correction (see Fig. 7.39c).

Strengthening the abdominal muscles

Strong abdominal muscles support the torso and can help to prevent or alleviate back pain. As discussed earlier in this chapter, one of the best exercises for safely working the abdominals is 'The Crunch.' (see Fig. 7.41). The crunch places the emphasis on the upper portion of the rectus abdominus; it should be accompanied by the 'Reverse Curl', which places the emphasis on the lower portion of the rectus abdominus. Together these two exercises ensure that you are working the abdominal area sufficiently.

The following exercises are designed to help you manage back trouble. It should be recognised, however, that these are only part of a wider approach to the problem. Learning how to lift correctly, stand, sit, and carry out other functional activities is vital if back pain is to be prevented or corrected. The ideal approach to back care

2. **Kyphosis:** Excessive curvature in the thoracic spine when viewed laterally (hunched back). In some cases, kyphosis may be congenital. It has also been associated with the development of osteoporosis. Stretching of the anterior shoulder muscles and stretching and strengthening of the posterior upper back muscles may be indicated (see Fig. 7.39b).

3. **Scoliosis:** Irregular lateral deviations in the spine form a posterior view in the sagittal plane. This can be caused by structural imbalances between the right and

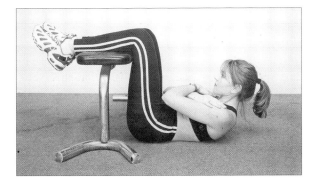

Figure 7.41: **The abdominal crunch.**

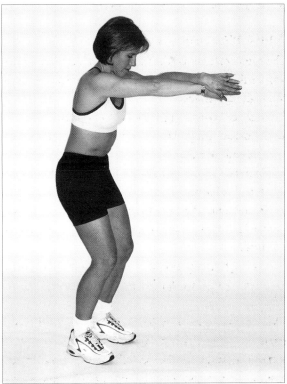

Figure 7.42: **Spine stretch (Rhomboids).**

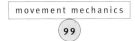

is a combined flexibility and strengthening program.

Those already suffering back problems should be advised to consult their doctor or physiotherapist, as exercise can aggravate certain types of back pain.

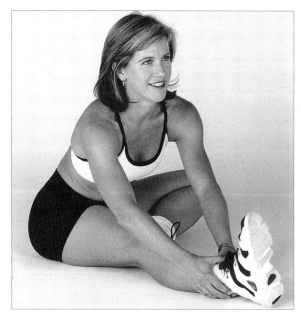

Figure 7.43: **Spine stretch.**

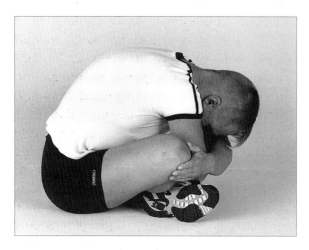

Figure 7.44: **Spine stretch.**

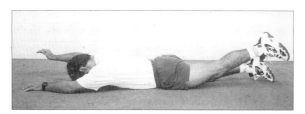

Figure 7.45: **Opposite arm/leg raise.**

Cervical spine or neck exercises: There are six basic movements of the neck — all these can be combined in a single stretch movement by bending the head forward, rotating to the side, then dropping the head back into extension, returning to the other side and finishing with the head on the chest. The direction can then be reversed.

Other neck stretches include tucking the chin and rotating the head (double chin exercise) and thrusting the neck forward and rotating the head (ostrich exercise). By resisting the movement of the neck with the palm of one or both hands one can perform isometric neck strengthening exercises.

Stretching and strengthening the back

The following exercises (see Figs 7.42–7.47) aim to improve and maintain maximum in the thoracic and lumbar regions of the spine. Many are also excellent for improving posture in general. When doing these stretches go to the point of mild discomfort, hold for 15–30 seconds then move into the stretch a little further.

- Spine stretch (1): Stretch hands above the head, 'think tall'.
- Spine stretch (2): Stand with partial knee flexion and reach forward with arms outstretched in the frontal horizontal position. Cross the forearms with palms together and reach forward. (see Fig. 7.42)
- Spine stretch (3): Move into a sitting position, reach forward, and clasp the hands behind the ankle. (see Fig. 7.43)
- Spine stretch (4): Now sit with legs crossed. Place the hands on opposite knees and pull. This will stretch the upper spine. (see Fig. 7.44)
- Shoulder stretch: Put right hand over right shoulder and left hand behind the back. Clasp fingers tightly and stretch, relax then repeat. Reverse arms and repeat the procedure.
- Opposite arm/leg raise: Lie prone on the floor and raise the opposite arm and leg slowly. Then repeat on the other side (see Fig. 7.45).
- Back arch: As above, except hands should be placed beside the body. As the head is raised, arms and shoulders should be stretched back (see Fig. 7.46).
- Spinal ligament stretch: Lying on the back with the hands behind the head, raise the head upwards and forwards.
- Abdominal and back extensor stretch: Lie supine

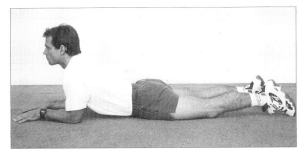

Figure 7.46: Back arch.

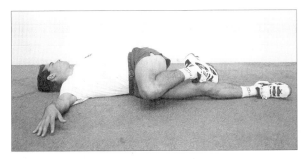

Figure 7.47: Spinal rotation.

Injury Recognition and Prevention

Prevention of injury is the Fitness Leader's first priority; however, being able to recognise that an injury has occurred is also of major importance. Some injuries are easily identified, others are not. Injuries due to physical activity fall into two broad categories:

Injury classification

1. Direct/extrinsic injury: Includes sudden traumatic injuries resulting from collision with some extrinsic (outside) force. Injuries such as bleeding, bruising (e.g. 'cork thigh'), bone fractures or breaks, dislocated joints and grade II to III ligament sprains are often caused by colliding with some object, an implement like a hand weight, or another person. Unsuitable environmental conditions like poor surface, damaged equipment or poor lighting can be causal to direct extrinsic injury.

2. Indirect/intrinsic (stress developed within the body): Includes overuse injuries that are divided into two sub-categories:

i) Acute overuse injury resulting in damage to soft tissue, from poor preparation for exercise; for example, inadequate warm-up and stretching that may result in a partial tear or rupture of the muscle-tendon unit or low grade ligament sprains.

ii) Chronic overuse injuries, which are often suffered by instructors and participants of exercise classes. Examples are: Achilles tendinitis, iliotibial band syndrome, Osgood Slater's disease, repetitive micro fatigue etc. There is also a secondary classification of chronic overuse injury, which results from poor initial diagnosis, or the mismanagement of a prior injury. Secondary overuse injuries are described as short- or long-term. Short-term injuries develop soon after the primary injury; for example, unrecognised or poor treatment of repetitive micro fatigue of the connective tissue of the anterior tibialis muscle may result in a stress fracture of bone. Long-term injuries develop years after the primary injury; for example, the development of a degenerative joint disease in an unstable joint that was a result of a sporting injury early in life.

(face up) on the floor with knees bent. Push the lower back into the floor while breathing out; then, while breathing in, arch the spine upwards.

🏃 Spinal rotation: Lying on the back, bend the right knee across the body and stretch the knee downwards with the left hand. Turn the head in the opposite direction (see Fig. 7.47).

🏃 Hip and knee flexion stretch: Bend one knee up towards the body while lying on the back. Hold and hug with the arms. Alternate legs.

🏃 Hip hitching: While lying prone, shorten one leg with respect to the other, then alternate legs.

🏃 Cat-arch back stretch: Crouching on all fours, raise the spine slowly upwards, then relax.

🏃 Alternate arm/leg stretch: While crouching on all fours, stretch the left hand above the head and right leg out behind, then alternate arms and legs.

Strengthening the back

This is best accomplished by doing controlled back hyperextensions. Suggested exercises include the opposite arm/leg raise, lifting the upper body only, or lifting the lower body only. When using a back extension machine on the gym floor, be careful to extend only to the neutral position and not into excessive hyperextension.

Defining injury terms

Pain is nature's way of telling us that something is wrong. The location and severity of the pain can often indicate the type of injury that has been sustained.

Muscle strain: A tear in the muscle-tendon complex. Muscle spasms are uncontrolled and painful muscle contractions that often occur as a protective mechanism after an injury has been sustained.

Ligament sprain: The principal function of ligaments is to maintain a joint's integrity while it is moving. Acute sprains of ligaments are graded as follows:
Grade I: Minor tearing of ligament fibres resulting in local tenderness, slight swelling and dysfunction, no joint instability.
Grade II: Partial tear of the ligament resulting in local tenderness, swelling, moderate disability and mild to moderate joint instability.
Grade III: Complete tear or rupture of the ligament causing strong tenderness, swelling and bruising with severe joint instability.

Tendinitis: An inflammation of the tendon sheath as a result of overuse or biomechanical inefficiency. Tennis elbow is often a result of tendinitis.

Haematoma: Although in the field of sports medicine haematomas generally refer to damage caused by a direct blow like a corked thigh, nearly all injuries to muscle result in the formation of a haematoma. Blood seeping from damaged blood vessels into surrounding tissue causes this. If there is bleeding in interstitial tissue, and if it becomes clotted in the area of the injury, a haematoma may develop. If left untreated a calcium deposit could form.

Stress fractures: Hairline breaks in a bone caused by overuse. If left unattended a shin splint can end up as a stress fracture to the tibia or fibula.

Bursitis: Bursae are closed sacs containing synovial fluid that are located in the body wherever there is a lot of friction and shock. Bursitis is an inflammation of the bursa.

Emergency First Aid for injury

The immediate treatment for almost all exercise-related injuries where the skin surface is not broken is the same, whether it is a pulled muscle, strained ligament, sore joint or a broken bone. The acronym for this 5-part program is RICED.

R = Rest: Rest is necessary because continued activity could extend the injury.

I = Ice: Ice decreases the bleeding from the injured blood vessels through vasoconstriction. Ice may be applied, for 15–20 minutes every 2–3 hours depending on the severity of the injury. Never use heat in the first 48 hours.

C = Compression: Compression limits the swelling which, if uncontrolled, could retard healing.

E = Elevation: Elevation of the injured part to above the level of the heart uses the force of gravity to help drain excess fluid.

D = Diagnosis: Consult a sports medicine specialist as soon as possible after the injury.

Remember: early treatment speeds recovery and a quick return to activity.

Exercise to Music

Aerobics to music was virtually unknown in the early '70s but it has become a very popular form of exercise.

The word 'aerobic' has been used for years in the scientific world to describe anything growing, living or occurring in the presence of oxygen. However, the term aerobics has become synonymous in the public mind with exercise to music.

An aerobic class has in fact become more than an aerobic program; it may also involve isolation strength work, flexibility, agility and coordination as well as providing a safe and social exercise environment.

Music

The choice of music is critical to the success of an exercise-to-music class. Music is made up of a series of beats arranged in regular rhythm patterns. The beat in music can be compared to a word in language. We can identify it and it can say something. Grouping beats together is like grouping words in a sentence, and putting groups of beats together is like forming a paragraph.

Beat: Like a musical word — a repetitive pulsing sound of music

Phrase: A musical sentence — a strong beat will signify the start of the phrase; this phrase will last 8 counts. A phrase is like a temporary musical idea.

Block: A musical paragraph — sometimes called a full phrase, indicating the completion of a musical idea. The block is made up of 32 counts (or four lots of 8 beats).

The block is the basic building unit for instructors, providing a framework for creating the aerobic class. Sometimes the regularity in the music temporarily changes. Such irregularities will require you to change the pattern of your moves to music.

Bridge: A musical exception to the rule: the bridge occurs where any group of beats does not complete a block of 32 counts, providing musical surprise.

Common bridges may be 2 beats, 4 beats, 8 beats, or 16 beats. Bridges can appear in any part of a song, but usually after a block in the verse, chorus, or instrumental.

Music Mapping

The process called Music Mapping is the written breakdown of music into an ordered arrangement of beats that allows you to understand the structure of the song. Knowing the landmarks of a song will assist you in cueing and moving your participants effectively as a whole.

Parts of a song for mapping

Introduction: A lead-in for the song, usually building in strength. Songs may simply start as a basic beat only.

Instrumental: Can be made up of a number of instruments together or solo. Generally instrumentals follow the melody of the song and commonly appear after a chorus.

Verse: The story of a song, which is generally sung, but may be spoken.

Chorus: The musical milestone, repeated often throughout a song to create familiarity.

Pre-chorus: This sits between the verse and chorus. It heralds the chorus and is also repeated like the chorus.

Break: The song breaks down to a bare minimum (such as a bass beat only). The sound is emptier, and provides a great place to introduce a new song when used in beat mixed tapes.

Loop: Just like an intro — signals the start of a song. Many songs have a loop to indicate the end. This may be a repeated chorus or a few lines from the chorus. It could be the main melody repeating constantly. Spotting this repetitive sound will allow you to pick the approaching end of the song.

Sound advice

Music speed plays an important role in determining i) success of teaching, ii) success of participants iii) safety in all class formats. Table 8.1 includes a recommended range of music speeds for different class types.

Class/Component	Beat Per Minute
Warm-Up	130-138 bpm
Low Impact	136-148 bpm
Mixed Impact	145-165 bpm
New Body	70-132 bpm
Muscle Conditioning	70-132 bpm
Interval(Work)	145-165 bpm
(X-high)	165-185 bpm
(Relief)	70-145 bpm
Step Reebok	118-122 bpm
Cool Down	120 bpm

The PITCH CONTROL can be used to alter speed of music. Remember that music speed may be reduced as well as increased.

Table 8.1: **Recommended beat ranges.**

Music selection

Music should be chosen for its ability to motivate, therefore choice will vary depending on clientele. Music should have a clearly defined, regular beat with a sense of urgency. It's important that the beat for the type of class is within the recommended range of beats per minute.

Teaching skills

Being an effective teacher takes much more than being in front of the class and executing some moves for others to follow. The difference between an average instructor and a great instructor is the ability to TEACH not just LEAD and to develop rapport with the class participants. You will need good vocal projection, a good teaching plan, music that helps not hinders and a clear idea of how to get the participants to do what you want them to!

How to Be a Great Instructor

- Don't say 'don't' — it tends to draw attention to the very thing the class is not meant to do.
- Use 'let's', 'we', 'your' and 'our' — it creates a team atmosphere.
- Establish and use eye contact with your class, to develop rapport.
- Avoid looking in the mirror, face the class when possible.
- Move around the room, to enable contact with everyone in the class.

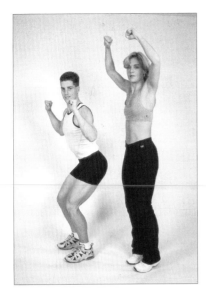

Figure 8.1: **Squat press.**

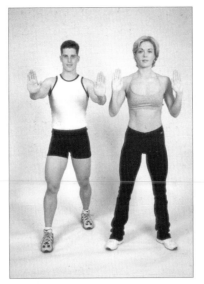

Figure 8.2: **Easy walk.**

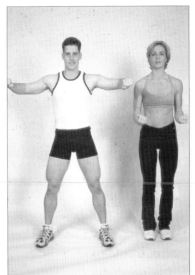

Figure 8.3: **Step touch.**

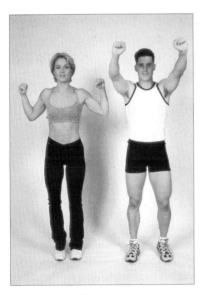

Figure 8.4: **Military press.**
(or arms up, overhead press).

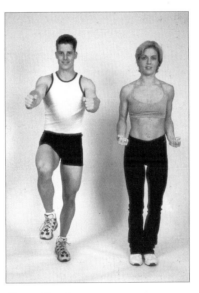

Figure 8.5: **Low row.**
(or: triceps side, triceps kickback).

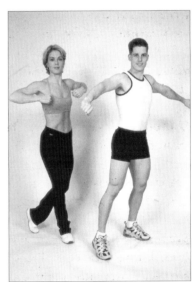

Figure 8.6: **Triceps press.**

🏃 Pay attention to first-timers, especially the ones at the back — they also need your help and attention.

🏃 Work on your form and exercise technique outside of the teaching situation.

Exercise vocabulary

Like resistance training, exercise to music has standard terms that are commonly used. It makes it much easier for instructors and participants alike if these terms are consistent (Figs. 8.1–8.6).

Mirror imaging

Mirror imaging is the practice of the instructor facing the class and directly imaging the participants. On the other hand, participant imaging is when the instructor faces the mirror and the participants follow the instructor from a posterior aspect.

Right footing

If the instructor starts teaching with his/her back to the class and they need to turn around, the skill of right

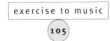

footing assures maintenance of a mirror image. In addition, it is also the skill of calling direction from the participant's point of view.

Successful Cueing

Making a group of people do the same thing at the same time is a tall order at the best of times. Instructors need to develop simple yet effective teaching techniques so that participants will be able to follow and understand instructions.

Developing the art of successful cueing is not only the identification of some simple teaching techniques, but learning how to combine and implement them for the greatest effect. In relation to a teaching style, remember that teaching style is not a predictor of success.

First things first

Before beginning to improve your teaching through cueing, you must first master the physical program. The physical routine should become second nature. Broaden exercise repertoire through varied activities including attending instructor training workshops, other instructors' classes, viewing videos, etc. Practise not only verbal commands but also interaction skills. As a general rule, spend 30% of practice time determining what you will be teaching (i.e. moves, combinations, etc) and 70% on how you will teach it (i.e. cueing — verbal/ non-verbal, learning curves, etc).

Cueing techniques

Instructors today are aware of the importance of the 'what, where, when and how' of verbal cueing. The cueing abilities of experienced instructors enable them to teach highly complex patterns and choreography to a class whilst maintaining a sense of achievement for all concerned.

It is interesting to note that participants receive 70% of their instruction non-verbally. Hence the importance of non-verbal cueing cannot be underestimated. Signs and symbols, facial expressions, correct technique and execution of movement by the instructor, music, props and suitable exercise selection are all methods of non-verbal cueing that can be used in a class.

Verbal cues

All verbal cues should be clear, concise and consistent with consideration to the following points:

Exercise identification (what): refers to the move that is to be performed. For example, upright row, step touch, easy walk.

Direction/placement (where): refers to the direction of the movement. For example, left, right, reverse or 'towards the door'.

Count-down/timing (when): refers to when the movement commences, how many repetitions to go and when to change.

Quality/technique (how): refers to the way in which the movement is to be performed.

Non-verbal cues

The aerobics instructor is the focal point of the class and as such, any move he/she does will be copied by the participants. It is critical therefore that all non-verbal cues are easily identified: Examples are:

- Signs or symbols
- Facial expression
- Music
- Body language
- Visual preview

Elements of effective cueing

Consistency: Develop a bank of easy-to-follow, easy-to-understand cues. Use them regularly.

Direct and to the point: Participants must be able to react to directions quickly and with confidence.

Good timing: Advance cues prepare participants for changes. Skills include count-down, logical exercise progression, using in-built music phrasing cues and easy-to-remember key words and symbols.

Be visible: Where you stand and how you position yourself (whether you are facing, or facing away from the class) can dramatically affect the impact of your cues.

Exercise selection: The progression from one exercise to another is a crucial element in effective cueing.

K.I.S. (Keep it Simple): Don't get carried away. Simplify what you do — too much often leads to mixed messages and techniques either working against one another or being used out of context.

Voice projection: Consider not only your projection but your tone and pitch.

Warm-ups

All phases of the aerobic workout are equally important in terms of developing the 'perfect end product'. Attention can be given to each component in order for it to reach its full potential, but this alone does not always lead to the desired outcome. Instructors realise that the success of one section of the workout is dependent on the success of the previous component, and this understanding highlights the increased importance of the warm-up.

The statement 'first impressions do count' holds true in the aerobic workout — whether it be an instructor's first class or just the beginning of each class.

The modern warm-up

When aerobics first came into vogue, very little attention was given to warming-up. Instructors and participants alike wanted to go straight into action and this resulted in unnecessary injuries. Fitness and health professionals around the world rallied and 'Thou Must Stretch' was the war-cry. Although safety was improved, instructors and participants found ten minutes of static stretching tedious and boring. Flexibility was only one ingredient of a warm-up and participants were not prepared physically or mentally for the workout.

The modern warm-up is dynamic and stimulating. The emphasis is on 'warming up' and 'mobility' and not on flexibility. Flexibility can be achieved in the cool-down by holding static stretches.

Integral components of a warm-up

The purpose of the warm-up is to prepare the body for the stress of overload during the conditioning phase of the class. Every warm-up must include the following:

Warming the body: By increasing body temperature the soft tissue (muscle and connective tissue) becomes more elastic, thus reducing the potential for strain. Blood flow also increases, thus enabling more oxygen and energy to be carried to the working parts of the body. The majority of the exercises in the warm-up should be brisk, rhythmical, compound movements. All muscle groups should be addressed.

Mobility: Many participants have compromised their posture prior to class by sitting or standing for long periods of time. This must be corrected and normal range of motion restored to ensure a safe and effective workout. Most of this will be achieved through the 'warming-up' exercises. However some areas of the body need special attention, such as the calves, hamstrings, lower back and hip flexors. Specific range-of-motion stretches should be included to target these important areas. This can be best achieved through dynamic stretching — repeating slow, controlled rhythmical movements, throughout the range of motion. Some static stretching can also be included to complement the dynamic stretching. This is particularly useful for new exercisers, as they can focus on alignment. In the end, instructors must also monitor the needs and wants of the exercising group to determine how much and what type of stretching is required.

Considerations for the warm-up

'You're on before you're on': It is important to welcome the participants, and introduce yourself. Following this, the group should be organised in the desired manner, the workout type confirmed and briefly outlined.

Music selection: The music type must suit the style of class, the participants, and carry with it a sense of urgency.

Speed: The speed of many modern warm-ups has increased slightly, with the acceptable range now being between 130 and 138 beats per minute.

Impact: Only low-impact moves should be included in the warm-up phase.

Range-of-motion stretches: These should be included in the warm-up phase to ensure adequate preparation for upcoming activities.

Complexity: Each group is different and the instructor must be able to adequately monitor their needs. The warm-up should be designed to prepare participants psychologically as well as physiologically.

Cool-downs

The cool-down of an aerobic class has two primary functions:

1. To return the body's physiological functions to a steady state and to assist the return of blood to the heart to prevent venous pooling.
2. To restore full range of motion and develop flexibility via stretching.

Phases of a cool-down

Recovery: Recovery after the conditioning phase is best accomplished by a continuation of the conditioning phase at a decreasing intensity. This can be carried out by performing rhythmical movements similar to those in the warm-up or by isolation floor exercises.

Flexibility: Flexibility work is essential at the conclusion of a class. Stretches should include all major muscle groups, with an emphasis on those most relevant to the workout.

Relaxation/education: While the areas above have a high priority, the cool-down period offers an opportunity for mental, emotional and physical relaxation. Further, it provides a chance to inform and educate the class participants and to encourage them with positive reinforcement.

Effective stretching during the cool-down

Every cool-down should include, as a minimum safety requirement, stretches for the major muscle groups used.

The cool-down section should account for at least 10% of the total class duration. In the case of classes for special populations, this component may account for up to 20% of the class time.

- 15 seconds is optimal time for holding a stretch.
- Create conducive conditions: dim the lights, use relaxing music with lowered volume, use a slower and softer instructor voice, and lower the air conditioning or turn the fans off.
- Stretching is enhanced by muscle relaxation. Therefore practices such as rubbing stretched muscles or applying self-massage should be encouraged.
- Effective stretching is only possible while a muscle is relaxed, therefore avoid bearing weight on the muscles being stretched.

Base Moves and Elements of Variation

Moves are the basic building blocks of all our programmes. The ability to classify base moves and then add variety by applying Elements of Variation is the first step towards creating a professional class.

Identifying Base Moves

In order to classify moves into appropriate categories, we must first break them down into their most basic form.

Elements of Variation

The acronym DR T LUMP is used to describe the Elements of Variation.

Direction: Refers to the aerobic room compass and where you want to go in the room.

Rhythm: Refers to changes in timing (slow/fast); e.g. from a step touch to dumbbell step touch.

Travel: Refers to the way you get to your destination on the aerobic room compass.

Levers: Refers to the limb length used; e.g. short lever/long lever.

Uni-lateral: Refers to the number of arms used in a move: uni = one arm, bi = two arms.

Mode: Refers to the intensity of a move; eg, non-impact, low-impact, high-impact.

Plane: Refers to arm lines/height in relation to the shoulders. Working in a hi-plane indicates working the arms above the shoulders, mid-plane at shoulder height and in a low-plane below the shoulders.

Low impact: is defined as a movement where one foot remains in contact with the ground most of the time.	Four low-impact moves: 1. Step touch 2. Touch step 3. Lift steps 4. Walking
High impact: is defined as any movement where both feet are off the ground at any point in time.	Four high-impact moves: 1. Running 2. Jumping 3. Hopping 4. Liftsteps
Non-impact: is defined as movement where both feet are in contact with the ground all of the time.	Three non-impact moves: 1. Lunges 2. Squats 3. Non-impact march

Table 8.2: **The base moves.**

Using these Elements of Variation the base moves can be expanded to give an unlimited supply of movement ideas and patterns (see Table 8.2).

Basic Learning Curves

Choreography can be defined as 'the art of planning and arranging movements to build a composition'. While choreography in the exercise class has gained popularity over recent years, the concept is still feared by many instructors. This fear can be cured by the application of 'learning curves' to the aerobic class.

Learning curves are teaching techniques that allow instructors to easily and effectively choreograph their exercise program. In addition, they also assist participants in mastering movement sequences/combinations, thereby maximising the efficiency and enjoyment of their workout.

Classification

Being able to classify learning curve techniques and labelling them adds a new dimension to instructor communication. For example, instructors can now be more specific when engaging in choreography exchange sessions or workshops as to the specific techniques used to arrive at the end product. Further, 'Log Book' summaries of workout sessions can now be more explicit, even though brief.

Linear progressions: Unlike combinations, linear progressions consist of a series of moves that link smoothly together and are not repeated in a predictable manner.

Pyramid: Repetitions of a move or sequence of moves are gradually increased.

Reverse pyramid: Repetitions of a move or sequence of moves are gradually reduced, leading to a more complex combination.

Pure repetition: A movement pattern or combination is taught, and learning occurs by repeating this total product over and over.

Add-on method: This is also referred to as the building block method. In essence it is another way of teaching part-to-whole but only one element at a time is added.

Link method: Another version of part-to-whole teaching. Moves A and B are taught and then linked together in a double move combination. The same is done for moves C and D; finally (A+B) and (C+D) are joined to develop a four-move combination.

Layer technique: A pattern that can be repeated is established. Changes to this pattern are gradually layered to obtain more value from the original concept.

Holding pattern addition: A number of moves are taught in a sequence and then a holding pattern/move is interspersed between sub-components. By adding this holding pattern the original length of the sequence is expanded.

Holding pattern removal: This technique is the reverse of that outlined above, whereby the sub-components of a combination are taught originally and a holding pattern is placed between them; this holding pattern is gradually removed to eventually arrive at the end product. The holding pattern provides a comfort zone when complex moves are being taught.

Association method: To assist the recall of exercises associate them with key words, numbers, or the sides of the room. This improves participant attention and provides an element of fun.

Organised action: (see page 110) Many teaching techniques may be used to make moves and classes successful, ranging from a simple follow-me approach through to more choreographic learning curves very specific to combinations. Regardless of the class type, even the simplest teaching technique can allow creativity and optimise the potential for all movement patterns. Two such applications that reinforce this are freestyle applications and the organised action format. The simplistic nature of each makes them an asset to an instructor's teaching skills.

Freestyle: A freestyle approach to aerobics classes focuses on a series of techniques for combining movement patterns in a simple 'follow-me' style, not necessarily emphasising any patterning to be recalled or repeated. The techniques used give the class a back-to-basics emphasis which allows any participant to focus on workout intensity.

Linear progression

Linear progression is the process by which a series of minor progressive adjustments are made to the move being performed, (e.g. progress through some moves by changing the arm line only, then change the leg pattern only, etc). By focusing at any stage during the linear progression, and adapting simple strategies, you can achieve a lot more from basic moves. Two strategies that may be used during the pause in the flow of linear progression are:

The zig-zag method: At any stage in the progression, pause and then back-track through the previous few movements in the reverse order, then repeat them in the original order and continue. Zig-zagging can be done more than once during the pause.

The top-and-tail method: At any stage in the linear progression, join two moves together and repeat them a number of times. Then add a new move to the tail of the progression and remove the initial move from the top. This now forms a new pair of moves and the same process can continue.

Organised Action

The number of moves available is not limitless, but the way moves are presented can be varied significantly. A great way to add variety to classes, using familiar moves in a different format, is to adopt a process of Organised Action. This concept is not new, but making the most of patterns utilised will keep intensity, interest, and effectiveness high, while creating a positive social atmosphere. Preparation is still the key to successful implementation. Some of the benefits of Organised Action are:

Variety: Common basic moves presented in a different format create interest. New travel patterns in groups move participants away from any territorial spots.

Value: Makes economical use of basic moves. Only a small number of moves are used at one time, and are repeated.

Instructor relief: The instructor's emphasis can shift from performing to organising and motivating the activities.

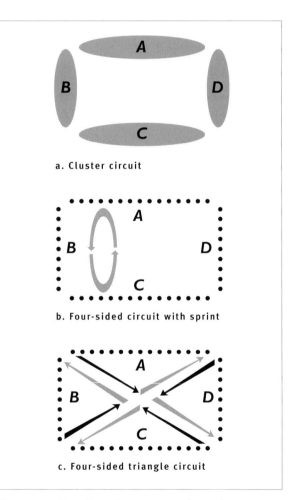

a. Cluster circuit

b. Four-sided circuit with sprint

c. Four-sided triangle circuit

Figure 8.7: **Sample perimeter group formations.**

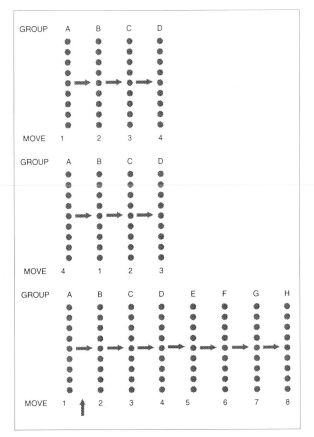

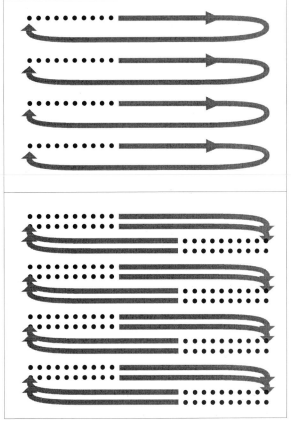

Figure 8.8: **Line circuits (top & middle) four line non rotating circuit, (bottom) eight line rotating circuit.**

Figure 8.9: **Relays: (top) single end relays, (bottom) double ended relay.**

Socialisation: A friendly and motivating atmosphere is developed in the organised class. This is again to the instructor's advantage.

To keep variety and success coming into your classes, choose grouping formats from the following Organised Action plans.

Perimeter groups (see Fig. 8.7)

🏃 Circle the class around the room to spread them out before dividing them into groups.

🏃 Try to make groups as even as possible.

🏃 Groups look to the right. When given the command 'change' they move to the right and do what that group was doing.

Variations

• More than four groups can be made.

• After all the groups have performed all the moves maintain the formation but give each group completely new moves.

Line circuits (see Fig. 8.8)

🏃 Give the entire group a holding move before organisation starts. Move entire group into a smaller space to make group-forming easier. Nominate four regular participants as line leaders.

🏃 Give each group a different move. Groups look to the line on their right for the next exercise.

🏃 On the command 'change' groups stay where they are and perform the new move.

🏃 Line D will not be able to see line A so the instructor must demonstrate their move.

Variations

• After all four moves have been completed by each group the moves can be joined together into a combination and, where applicable, travelled.

Relays (see Fig. 8.9)

🏃 Divide the class into groups and perform a holding move.

🏃 First person in each group runs/walks to the other

end and back. Upon return they tag the next person and move to the end of the line.

🏃 The instructor regularly changes the holding move.

🏃 Caution participants on the danger of travelling or turning too quickly. Avoid competition, as this can over-motivate or become a turn-off for some participants. Do not allow the relay runner to touch the wall or floor before turning.

Variations

• Upon reaching the far end the relay runner performs an exercise, e.g. four astride jumps.

• Have a half-way station so that an exercise is performed half way down then another at the end.

• Pick-a-Card — have cards with the name of common exercises in a box at the far end. Participants run to the end, select a card and perform the exercise as described. For novelty throw in a fun exercise, e.g. dead ant.

• Props (balloons, bean bags, oranges) or themes (Christmas, Halloween, country & western) work well with relays.

Facing lines (see Fig. 8.10)

🏃 In this formation the facing groups can either move to the centre and back as in Fig. 8.10, or they can cross over completely as in diagram.

🏃 For larger classes make two or more sets of facing lines.

🏃 This can be combined with partner work. When crossing over always instruct participants which shoulder to pass by, e.g. R shoulder to R shoulder.

Cast-offs (see Fig. 8.11)

🏃 Instruct each group that they will be walking to the front of the line, turning to the right, walking to the far end and returning to their original position.

🏃 Vary the holding move between each cast-off and vary the direction participants will turn.

🏃 Ensure that all participants walk to the front of the line before turning.

🏃 Jogging can also be used, but it is best that the entire group moves at the same speed.

Variations

• The two outside groups walk down between the two inside groups; the two inside groups then walk out around the outside groups.

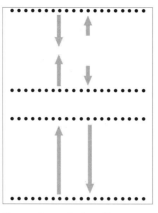

Figure 8.10: **Facing lines.**

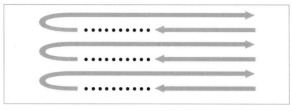

Figure 8.11: **Cast-offs.**

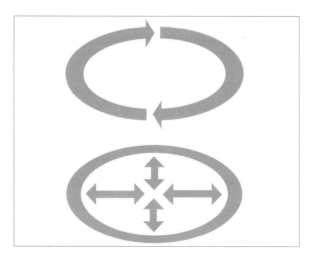

Figure 8.12: **Circles (top) basic circles (bottom) in and out.**

• Continuous cast-offs. Do not break up the walks with a holding move. As soon as the groups return after turning to the right they immediately turn and walk to the left.

Basic circles (see Fig. 8.12)

When walking/running in a circle it is important that the direction is changed regularly. Do not just call out 'change' — half the class will turn and the rest will keep going. There are better ways to change direction:

- While the group is travelling, warn them they are going to stop. Perform a holding move on the spot then signal travel in the opposite direction.
- From the outset, instruct the group they will take a set number of steps in each direction.
- Instructor joins the circle and peels the line diagonally across the room and continues in the opposite direction.
- Use gestures to signal the direction to be travelled. Use the 'stop' sign to warn of holding or direction change.

Snakes

- Lead into these patterns from a circle. These can be useful to change the direction of the circle.
- Simple race walking or jogging can be done for the entire snake or change the movement after turning at the end of every line.
- Instruct the class not to change moves until they get to the end of the line.

Major positional exercises

A list of exercises, by no means complete, for the four primary body positions is shown in Table 8.3. They are non-equipment variations only.

Classes Using Light Weights

Approximately half of the research studies conducted have shown that there is a significant difference in energy cost of exercise between exercising with or without hand weights. To significantly increase energy cost, exercises for the upper body need to be performed with an increased range of motion rather than an increased tempo of movement. Obviously there is a limit to the amount of arm movements that can be performed.

Position	Basic Exercise	Common Variations	
Standing	Lunge	Front Back	Side
	Squat	Wide	Narrow
	Heel raise	Wide Narrow	Unilateral Bilateral
	Balanced	Free leg abduction/adduction Toe touching Inward & outward hip rotation Flexion/extension/ hyperextension	
Prone	Push-up	Wide, narrow Staggered, extended	
	Rear lateral raises	Kneeling Lying	
	Hip extension	Kneeling Lying	
	Back extension	With lateral flexion	
Supine	Crunch	Full	Staggered stages
		Pulsing	Rotation/ twisting
	Reverse crunch	Heels close to gluteals Legs extended to ceiling	Feet on floor
	Lateral flexion	Short reach Long reach	
	Reverse push-up	Elbows wide Elbows close to ribs	
	Hip extension	One leg extended Both feet grounded	
	Dips	Legs extended Heels close to pelvis	
Side lying	Hip/leg abduction	Straight leg	
	Hip/leg rotation	Outward Inward	
	Hip/leg extension	Shoulder adduction	
	Oblique crunch	Unilateral Lateral	With rotation
	Side push-up		

Table 8.3: **Exercises for the four primary body positions.**

Selection guide

1. **Weight selection:** In order to prevent excessive overload of the deltoids, recommended weight selections are:

	Female	Male
Beginners	0 to ½ kg	½ to 1 kg
Intermediate	½ to 1 kg	1 to 1½ kg
Advanced	1 to 1½ kg	1½ to 3 kg

2. Music selection: Speed of music will vary according to weight size, lever length, ROM and stationary versus travelling moves. As a general rule the following bpms are recommended:

    70–115 bpm for strength moves

    120–130 bpm for stationary moves

    120–132 bpm for travelling moves

3. Lever length: Incorporate a mixture of long and short levers and ensure appropriate bpm's are used.

- Long lever work may be performed at slower speeds (e.g. half time).
- Avoid building of momentum as the risk to the joints and the muscle is increased.

Two examples of classes using weights are described below:

1. The Body Sculpt Class

Body Sculpt is a class specially designed to condition all muscle groups by utilising hand weights or other resistance equipment. The main objective of the class is to improve muscular strength and endurance.

A Body Sculpt class is typically slower and more stationary than a New Body class, with music speed ranging between 70–132 bpm. The level of resistance should be appropriate for each individual participant, the upper level being 5 kg.

Technical definition: Movements are executed with resistance provided by a combination of body weight, hand weights, rubberised bands and step to improve muscle strength and endurance. Techniques such a blitzing, pyramiding/reverse pyramiding, negative reps, pre-exhaustion and super sets can be used to gain the most from this class.

Fitness level: All.

Music speed: 70–132 bpm.

Equipment: The level of resistance should be appropriate for each individual participant, the upper limit being 3 kg.

Special considerations: Muscle groups are targeted for overall balance.

Consumer definition: Condition your muscles with a variety of standing and floor exercises using body weight, hand weights, rubberised bands and step. Movements are slow and controlled to achieve muscle strength and endurance and the amount of coordination that is required is minimal. The class has no aerobic work but is a good addition to your aerobic program.

Client considerations: There are essentially two types of clients who are attracted to Sculpt classes:

1. The hard core enthusiasts who generally want to overload each muscle group until it is fatigued.
2. The soft-core enthusiast who wishes to work all body parts in a format more like a stretch-and-tone class with light hand weights.

Since both types of clients may exist in the one centre, the focus of one Sculpt class to the next may need to change. Additionally, the focus in one class may need to be adapted for both types of client.

Muscle balance and sequencing:

When developing movement choreography for a Sculpt class it is important to consider the appropriate balance of muscle groups and in what order muscles should be targeted. Balancing opposing muscle groups is important to prevent injuries and to maintain correct posture. Both agonist and antagonist muscle groups should be worked, while considering postural and phasic muscles. When linking two or more moves together, consider not only which muscles are being worked, but the physiological and biomechanical stresses placed on the muscles and joints. Beware of overworking any one muscle group. It would seem obvious to target large muscle before smaller muscles, and phasic muscles before postural.

2. The New Body workout

The New Body workout is a valid and very popular exercise-to-music class taught in most fitness centres throughout Australia. Primarily it incorporates a number of endurance-based upper body exercises executed with light hand held weights (½ kg to 2 kg). The energy cost of this class is maintained by incorporating non-impact or low-impact movements.

Technical definition: This workout incorporates upper body exercises with light hand held weights which are performed in association with non-impact and low impact aerobic moves.

Fitness levels: All.

Music speed: 70–132 bpm.

Equipment: Weights should be no heavier than 2 kg.

Considerations: Weights should be utilised for a minimum of 50% of the class duration.

Consumer definition: New Body combines upper body exercises with light hand weights and easy-to-follow low-impact moves. This class has no running or jumping. The result is a lower intensity workout that is maintained for an extended period to enable calorie burning and muscle conditioning. This workout can be adapted for all fitness levels and the specific upper body conditioning is a great reason to add it to your existing fitness program.

Physiology and the New Body class: The reduction in fat stores that participants may have noticed from a New Body class is due to a number of factors:

1. Increased energy expenditure may be due to more classes being done per week, or the fact that participants are performing movements correctly.
2. A decreased exercise intensity, coupled with an increase in duration, enhances the oxidation of fat stores within the body.
3. By working at a lower exercise intensity (60–70% max. HR) the percentage of fat metabolised for energy (work) is greater than that at a higher intensity (70–85% max. HR). However as energy expenditure is lower, exercise duration must be increased to enable participants to experience a reduction in body fat. Hence in a New Body class a minimum of 4 minutes at a steady state of 60–70% max. HR is maintained to enable this increased fat utilisation to occur.

Additionally it should be noted that the use of hand-held weights provides for an increase in muscular strength and endurance and, when combined with low impact movements, improves cardiovascular fitness.

Guidelines for Running Aerobic Classes

❋ The class must include a warm-up phase (5–10 minutes), a conditioning phase (at least 20 minutes) and a cool-down phase (5–10 minutes).

❋ Music should be selected to allow for a good general warm-up at a gentle rate before more strenuous work is carried out.

❋ Entry into the class should be discouraged after the warm-up has started.

❋ Well-cushioned supportive shoes should be compulsory.

❋ Participants should be encouraged to attend exercise classes or carry out some other form of aerobic exercise at least 3 days a week.

❋ As far as possible classes should be structured to cater at least for beginning and advanced exercisers (preferably with an intermediate level), with separate classes conducted for each.

❋ Stretching in the cool-down should be static or PNF and should include the major muscle groups used in the exercise class.

❋ All new participants in a class should be questioned as to their previous exercise levels and advised as to the level recommended for their purpose.

❋ Participants should be advised from the start of the program as to how long the class will be, and of any idiosyncrasies of the class that may not be expected.

❋ Participants must be asked if they are taking any form of medication. Where no knowledge about a medication is immediately available, steps should be taken to ascertain contraindications of exercise, if any.

❋ Participants should be advised to exercise before rather that after eating, but that limited non-alcoholic fluid intake before (and even during) extended exercise is advisable.

❋ Exercise involving deep knee bends, forward flexion or hyperextension of the lower back should be avoided.

❋ Attention must be given to the correct procedures in carrying out exercises, eg. sit-ups should be done with legs bent, leg raises with some back support, etc.

❋ Advice should be given to certain participants about the level of difficulty of some exercises, eg. many men may have difficulty with certain flexibility exercises more suited to women (adductor/abductor stretches, back flexes, etc.).

❋ Precaution must be taken at all times to prevent both acute and chronic injury.

❋ Ideally, one other instructor should be on the floor assisting the instructor taking the class. His/her job is to correct exercises and give advice and encouragement, particularly for beginners.

❋ Participants should be asked to remove watches, jewellery and other accessories that may interfere with the full range of movement of an exercise.

❋ Clothing should be loose-fitting to allow proper freedom of movement.

❋ Ballistic type stretching is not advisable.

❋ Instructors should have a current first aid certificate including knowledge of cardiopulmonary resuscitation (CPR). A good first aid kit and instant ice packs should also be readily available in the unlikely event of an accident. An emergency phone number should also be close by.

❋ Floor areas should not be overcrowded. Crowding restricts the range of exercises that can be carried out and makes running difficult, if not dangerous.

❋ Ensure the exercise space is well ventilated and try to keep the temperature relatively cool, at between 15–20°C. Cold air from an air conditioner or open window should be avoided.

Aquafitness

Aquafitness (sometimes called 'Waterobics', 'Aquarobics', 'Hydro-exercise' etc.) is a rapidly growing mode of exercise based on a wide variety of exercises, games, circuits and dances that are performed in water. Many people join aquafitness programs not only to improve fitness but to meet others, to learn something new, to regain confidence after illness, or simply to experience an enjoyable activity. Anyone can join an Aquafitness program, including non-swimmers. Its popularity is assured because it is an exercise activity suitable for a wide range of people, whether young or old, able or disabled, fit or unfit.

While performing exercises in water participants deal with forces that are not experienced on land. These are:

1. Propulsive forces: There are two primary propulsive forces that move swimmers, through water — propulsive lift and propulsive drag. Since propulsive forces are rarely used in aqua classes they will not be discussed further here.

2. Resistive drag force: These forces oppose forward motion and are divided into three classifications a) profile drag b) surface or skin friction drag and c) wave drag. Profile drag is the most significant type of drag experienced when moving in water and is therefore of primary importance to the aqua instructor. Profile drag occurs in direct opposition to forward movement and is exploited in aquafitness classes to provide overload for the working muscles. The amount of profile drag created depends upon the overall shape and size of the body or body part and the speed at which it moves through the water.

3. Buoyancy: This is a force that opposes the effects of gravity. The rule that determines whether a body will float or sink is called Archimedes' Principle. This states that a body that is partially immersed in a fluid will experience an upward buoyant force that is equal to the volume of fluid displaced by the body. Overall body density and the amount of air contained in the lungs determine buoyancy.

This principle is important when applied to Aqua. Participants vary in density and therefore will float to differing degrees. The overweight participant may have a tendency towards floating (due to an increase in fat mass), whilst the leaner participant (with less fat mass) may find floating difficult.

Benefits

The benefits of exercising in water have been well known since Greek and Roman times. Examples are:

1. Exercising in water is easier: it supports body weight (up to 85% in water up to chest level).
2. Water acts as a shock absorber, reducing stress on joints.
3. Water provides resistance to motion through resistive drag. The intensity of the exercise can be easily controlled by varying the degree of resistance (drag). The amount of drag experienced depends on the size and shape of an object or body part as well as the speed at which it is moved through water. By moving faster, or in deeper water where the resistance is greater, the intensity is increased. By moving more slowly or in shallower water the intensity is decreased.
4. Water acts as a coolant to prevent overheating (provided the water temperature is not too high).
5. Water allows a full range of movement without excessive strain. Less coordinated individuals can carry out movements in water without the embarrassment they may feel with exposed land-based classes.
6. There is little post-exercise stiffness. This is due, possibly, to the lack of eccentric muscular contractions when using water as a mode of resistance.
7. The massaging effect of water increases circulation and promotes relaxation.
8. Aquafitness is a novel and enjoyable way to become and stay fit.
9. Buoyancy properties of water assist in supporting the body (up to 90%), often making exercise feel easier.
10. Up to 85% of jarring is eliminated as the water absorbs impact when jogging or jumping.
11. Those with sporting injuries can still exercise in water. They need not lose overall fitness during rehabilitation from injury.
12. Many of the exercises can be done in pairs or groups and this type of activity encourages socialisation and the overall fun of the program.
13. Participating in an Aquafitness program will assist non-swimmers in gaining water confidence (initially they can wear buoyancy vests).

Safety Factors

Some important safety considerations are:

1. A momentary rise in blood pressure occurs when a person enters the water, therefore immersion should be gradual.
2. There is a risk of hypothermia if body heat is lost too quickly during or immediately following exercise in pools with a temperature below 25^0 C, and a risk of hyperthermia where the temperature is above 30^0 C.
3. Pool chemicals should be maintained at strictly correct levels to prevent the risk of infection or skin irritation. Showering and using moisturiser after the class are recommended, as is the use of antifungal powder on the feet.
4. Teaching correct form is essential as close individual monitoring of an aquafitness class is difficult, e.g.:
    • Avoid the natural inclination to jog and jump on the toes whilst in the water. Use the whole foot in order to avoid cramp or leg injury.
    • Whenever performing stomach-strengthening exercises with the back against the pool wall, be sure the pelvis is tilted forward.
5. When demonstrating on the poolside, wear adequate protective footwear or use a gym mat, etc.
6. Where possible, use non-verbal communication to save vocal cords.
7. Knowledge of First Aid, cardiopulmonary resuscitation and water rescue techniques is essential.

Venue Requirements

The following should be available in a good venue:
*   Correct depth of water, waist to chest deep.
*   Correct water temperature
*   25°C Aquarobics
*   28°C Pre- and post-natal

- 33°C Stretch and movement
- Non-slip pool surrounds and floor.
- Ramp or steps for entry and exit.
- A rail, ledge or gutter at water level.
- Sufficient areas around the pool for the instructor to demonstrate.

Programming for Aquafitness

Aquafitness classes should follow the same general guidelines as any other program. The class should include a warm-up, conditioning and cool-down phase, keeping in mind that within these parameters there are a number of variables that can be changed, such as the depth of water, the speed of the exercises or the amount of turbulance created. The instructor can also use different kinds of music and equipment (leg/arm fins, balls, hoops, inner tubes, flippers etc.) to add variety.

Target Groups

One main benefit of an Aquafitness program is that all age groups and fitness levels can participate. Some of the groups for whom the activity is suitable are:
- Athletes in training
- Injured athletes
- Children
- Pre and post-natal women
- Overweight people
- Older adults
- Frail aged
- Disabled — physically and intellectually

Guidelines for some of these groups are considered below. General guidelines for the running of Aquafitness classes are given at the end of the chapter.

Athletes

Aquafitness can be an excellent alternative activity for very fit people or athletes nursing an injury. Circuit formats, i.e. exercise stations placed around the pool, can provide an intensive cardiovascular workout. Programs for athletes are usually planned specifically to improve performance in a particular sport or activity. Some of their special needs are considered below.

Profile of the athlete:
- High aerobic fitness
- Good muscle tone/strength
- Motivated
- Often poor flexibility
- Co-ordination could be improved
- Often stressed.

Guidelines:
1. Capitalise on the resistance properties of water. Include hand-boards, weights and flotation devices.
2. Use deepwater techniques to increase difficulty and aerobic effect.
3. Include circuit training.
4. Work on flexibility and co-ordination.
5. Encourage relaxation.

Children

Programs for children are often run as part of the school curriculum these days. The objective may be to build water confidence as part of a learn-to-swim program or as an alternative to competitive sport, with the emphasis on social development and learning through play.

Under-12-years profile:
- High lean tissue/fat ratio causes children to lose body heat rapidly.
- Able to perform tasks suited to their stage of development.
- Can be at various levels of water confidence.

Guidelines:
1. Water should be heated (25° C).
2. Water should be no deeper than chest height.
3. Exercises should be simple to understand, short in duration, and fun.
4. Add variety by including equipment in class (e.g. hoops, rings, balls, inner tubes, etc.).
5. Exercises can include simple variations on themes of movement, including:
- Walking in circles
- Jumping-jacks
- Bunny hops
- Marching
- Jogging

🏃 Dancing

🏃 Hopping

🏃 Games

Pre-natal Women

Pregnant women can benefit enormously from an aqua program. Exercising on land during pregnancy can be awkward, whereas in the water it is very comfortable. Special considerations are a doctor's clearance and avoiding heated pools in the early stages of pregnancy. In fact, many doctors recommend aquafitness classes for pregnant women because in water their condition or extra size does not disadvantage them. When prescribing such a program it is important to remember that pregnancy is a healthy state, not a 'medical condition'!

Profile of the pre-and post-natal woman:

- Increased heart rate and cardiac output.
- Increased core temperature.
- Increased breast size may lead to fibrous tissue breakdown, which is irreversible.
- A special hormone, 'relaxin', is released to loosen the joints in the pelvic area. This can have a weakening effect on joints.
- Postural changes can lead to lower back pain if care is not taken.
- In about 30% of women the linea alba between the rectus abdominus muscles may soften and weaken.
- About 30% of women who have never had children and 80% of pregnant women experience a weakening of pelvic floor muscles, which can cause incontinence.
- As pregnancy progresses, circulation in the lower limbs becomes impaired, often leading to severe cramping.

Guidelines:

1. Check on the participant's general amount of exercise undertaken during pregnancy.
2. Work at a maximum level of 140 bpm.
3. Avoid overheated pools (over 30⁰ C) for pre-natal classes.
4. Adequate breast support is essential during exercise.
5. Key skeletal muscles should be strengthened to compensate for the change in centre of gravity: in particular, abdominals, gluteals, hip flexors, exten-

sors of the spine and neck.

6. Check for separation between the abdominal muscles by placing fingers between the bands of recti muscles when the woman is lying in the supine position with chin raised. Three or more fingers' width indicates a need for a gentle abdomen-strengthening program.
7. Include pelvic floor exercises.
8. Avoid exercises involving toe pointing as these can precipitate leg cramp. Add exercises to increase circulation in lower limbs, such as calf stretch, ankle circles, etc.
9. Advise pregnant participants to eat complex carbohydrate 1 hour prior to a class in order to avoid fatigue and dizziness. Encourage a well-balanced diet.

Older Adults

Much of the growth in popularity of aquafitness classes has been due to the interest of older adults who find such classes fun, easy to do, and not physically stressful on aged joints. People over 50 are often the most loyal, highly motivated and consistent participants in aquafitness classes. They have few restrictions on their time, such as careers or dependent families, and they are usually overjoyed to find an exercise activity they can do safely.

Profile of the older adult:

- Often have weak muscles.
- A tightening of postural muscles and weakening of phasic muscles with age can lead to increased lower back problems.
- Freedom of movement can be restricted due to joint deterioration and swelling caused by arthritis.
- Poor diet, malabsorption of nutrients and changes in hormone levels can lead to brittle bones.
- Gradual loss of proprioceptive sensitivity in the feet affects sense of position, balance and body awareness. Around 60% of older women may have weak pelvic floor muscles which can affect bladder control, causing incontinence.
- Possible heart and circulatory disorders.
- Often on medication.

Guidelines:

1. Focus on gentle exercise.
2. Ensure water temperature is 28–33°C.

3. Focus on body awareness, balance, co-ordination, flexibility and strength.
4. Avoid grinding, repetitive movements that can cause injury.
5. Include pelvic floor exercises.
7. Teach heart rate monitoring and its purpose (use radial not carotid pulse).
8. Discourage participants with heart conditions from exercising with their arms above their heads.
9. Check medication and its effect during exercise.

Aquafitness Exercises

The following figures illustrate body positions, stretches, and exercises that are used in the water. Others can be adapted from those used on land.

Body Positions

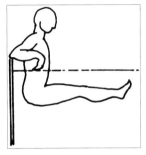
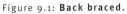

Figure 9.1: **Back braced.**

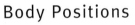

Figure 9.2: **Sit float.**

Stretches

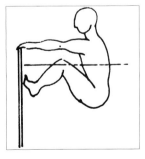

Figure 9.3: **Backstroke start.**

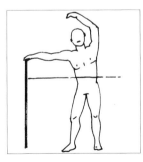

Figure 9.4: **Side stretch.**

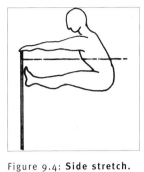

Figure 9.5: **Quad stretch.**

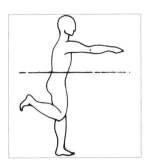

Figure 9.4: **Side stretch.**

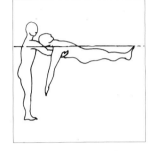

Figure 9.6: **Universal stretch (hamstring, back, shoulders).**

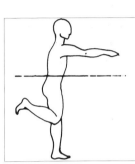

Figure 9.7: **Partner floats**

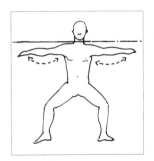

Figure 9.8: **Backward and forward flyes.**

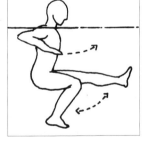

Figure 9.9: **Breast stroke arms, cossack legs.**

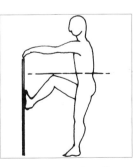

Figure 9.10: **Pool wall step-ups.**

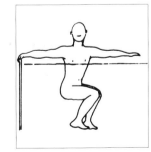

Figure 9.11: **Side tucks.**

Exercises

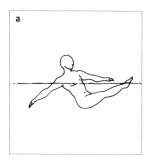

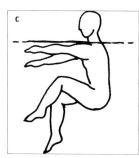

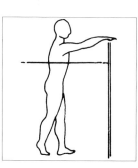

Fig. 9.14: Front lean flat-footed backward kicks (alternate feet 15 cm off pool floor).

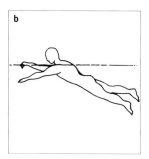

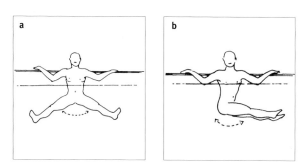

Figure 9.12a, b & c: Water burpies (leg extensions, knee tucks, backwards kicks).

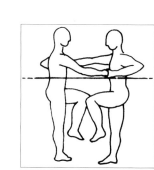

Fig. 9.15: Washing machine jog.

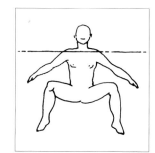

Fig. 9.16: Tuck jumps.

Figure 9.13a & b: Back braced scissors.

Guidelines for Running Aquafitness Classes

The following are general guidelines for running Aquafitness classes:

🏃 Don't enter or leave the water abruptly. This can cause rapid changes in blood pressure, which may be dangerous in some people.

🏃 Don't exercise with the head under water or while holding the breath.

🏃 Where possible ensure there is protection if the bottom of the pool is slippery. Old sandshoes with holes cut in them to let the water out can be useful.

🏃 Avoid exercises involving excessive extension of the lower back, particularly while using the poolside for support.

🏃 Avoid using overheated pools (over 30^0 C) for general exercise classes, as they can cause a build-up of heat in the body (stretch and movement classes, however, may be carried out in temperatures up to 33^0 C).

🏃 Warm-up and cool-down gradually, as in all exercise classes. When starting, include exercises to increase circulation to the lower legs and feet.

🏃 Ensure that all participants can swim or are sufficiently confident, at least, in water. Inability to swim should not exclude a person from participating, but instructors ought to be aware of individuals' limitations.

🏃 Remember that showering and using skin moisturiser and anti-fungal powder on the feet is recommended after water classes.

🏃 Close attention should be paid to participants at all times to ensure that no one is getting cold, tired or in any way distressed.

🏃 Instructors should be aware of the environment in which they are working, e.g. who is responsible for providing emergency services, where the telephone is located, etc., and have a detailed knowledge of cardiopulmonary resuscitation, water rescue techniques and First Aid.

Fitness Testing

Traditionally fitness assessments have been performed as a collection of specific fitness tests designed to assess several physiological constructs. It may be commendable to ensure all bases are covered, but does this traditional approach benefit the trainer and client? For example, if an individual wishes to improve his/her cardiovascular fitness, is strength testing appropriate? It is important to select tests that are relevant to the client's fitness objectives. Fitness Leaders should develop a fitness testing toolbox that can be tailored individually to match each client's needs. This allows him/her to individually or collectively assess constructs such as blood pressure, resting heart rate, body mass, height, body composition, body fat distribution, cardiorespiratory function, flexibility and muscular strength, power and endurance.

In this chapter basic health-related fitness testing protocols will be considered. More complex laboratory-based tests used to assess constructs such as cardiac function and electromyography should only be carried out under strictly controlled conditions and performed by suitably qualified personnel.

When selecting fitness tests for clients the following should be considered:

- Select tests that suit the cross section of the population with whom you work.
- Select tests that are non-threatening.
- Select tests that provide relevant information to the tester and to the person being tested.
- Select tests that are motivational.
- Select tests that provide practical baseline information and, where possible, have comparison tables.
- Select tests that are valid.
- Select tests that are reliable and easily repeatable.
- Select tests that do not require technical or medical supervision.

Evaluation

Evaluating a client's health and fitness status is not something that should be taken lightly, as many people are apprehensive about being put through a physical assessment. Bearing this in mind, the instructor should endeavour to adapt the tests to the specific needs of the client.

When selecting tests of any type, accuracy is a major priority. All tests selected should be:

Valid: A test is considered valid if it measures what it is supposed to. For example, body weight is a valid measure of overall body mass and level of hydration, but it is an invalid measure of body composition. If a test is not valid consider it useless.

Reliable: Reliability refers to how accurately a test measures the same construct on repeated occasions.

Sensitive: This describes the degree to which a particular test can detect small changes, for example, a VO_2 max test performed using a gas analyser is a more sensitive test of cardiorespiratory function than an estimated submaximal VO_2 field test.

Pre-test Screening

Fitness testing is a form of physical examination. It usually involves physical activity, hence the question often asked is 'Can it be dangerous?'

Famous Swedish exercise physiologist Per Olaf Astrand says:

'The question is frequently raised whether a medical examination is advisable before commencing a training program. Certainly anyone who is doubtful about his/her state of health should consult a physician. In principle, however, there is less risk in activity than in continuous inactivity. In fact, it is probably more advisable to undergo a medical examination if one intends to be sedentary in order to establish whether one's state of health is good enough to stand the inactivity.'

For those under 35 years of age, with no obvious health risk (e.g. high blood pressure, a history of heart disease, overweight, diabetes mellitus), baseline fitness test results can serve as comparison data to assess future progress and serve as a motivational tool. For others it might be useful as a screening device, and to help devise a program to suit special needs.

Figure 10.1 is a simple screening test for determining the need for a medical clearance prior to being prescribed an exercise program.

Anyone scoring 5 or more points on the scale should be comprehensively screened by a suitably qualified person before beginning exercise. Those scoring under 5 who are apparently healthy can begin a graded exercise program without further testing.

The Exercise Safety Questionnaire (Fig. 10.2) is an example of how a comprehensive lifestyle-screening questionnaire can be adapted to the specific needs of the fitness industry. The relevant lifestyle questions have been summarised into eight sentences and the client is only asked to give a yes or no to each question. If the client answers 'yes' or 'not sure' to any question, then the instructor discusses the matter further and recommends that the client gets medical advice and clearance before beginning an exercise program (see also Fig. 4.4).

Age:	Score
under 35	0
35–44	1
45–54	2
55 & over	4
Obesity level:	
Normal weight	0
More than 20% overweight	2
Waist to hip ratio greater than 0.9	3
Blood pressure:	
under 140/90	0
under 160/95	2
over 160/95	4
not known	2
Medical history:	
previous cardiac trouble	6
diabetes mellitus	5
heart disease in family	2
heavy smoking (more than 10 day)	2
previously inactive	1
pregnant	5
lower back pain	5
Total:	
Score greater than 5: Comprehensive Lifestyle Screen Score less than 5: Commence a graded exercise program	

Figure 10.1: **Sample pre-test screening questionnaire.**

<table>
<tr><td colspan="3">

EXERCISE SAFETY QUESTIONNAIRE
Please check with your doctor or specialist before exercising

</td></tr>
</table>

For Your Safety: Please answer the following questions by ticking the appropriate box, and read the exercise advice below.

Tick to answer ✔	No	Yes or not sure
1. Have you ever had any injury, illness, back or joint condition that may be aggravated by vigorous exercise?	❏	❏
2. Have you ever had: Arthritis, Asthma, Diabetes, Epilepsy, Hernia, Dizziness, Gout, Circulation problems or an Ulcer?	❏	❏
3. Have you ever had a Heart condition, High Blood Pressure, Rheumatic Fever, Stroke, High Cholesterol, Palpitations, Murmurs or Pains in the chest?	❏	❏
4. Have your mother, father, brother or sister had any heart problems prior to age 60?	❏	❏
5. Are you now or have recently been pregnant?	❏	❏
6. Are you taking any prescribed medication?	❏	❏
7. Is there any other condition that might be reason to modify your exercise program?	❏	❏
8. Have you been doing regular vigorous exercise lately? If YES, what type of exercise?	❏	❏

BEGINNERS: Work at a slow pace and learn how to do each exercise correctly.
On each visit you will be able to work a little harder. Please ask your instructor for guidance.

Name:

Address: Postcode:

Employer: Work Phone:

How would you describe your current physical condition?

❏ Unwell   ❏ Overweight   ❏ Unfit   ❏ Healthy   ❏ Fit

What are the main benefits that you want from exercise?

❏ Fat loss   ❏ Improve Fitness   ❏ Increase size   ❏ Enjoyment

❏ Muscle tone   ❏ Maintain Fitness   ❏ Sport training   ❏ Good health

To improve your fitness, exercise at least 3 times per week. Fitness assessments are recommended to help you start safely and to monitor your progress. If you need advice or assistance any staff member will be glad to help you.

How did you find out about our Club?

I have completed the EXERCISE SAFETY QUESTIONNAIRE and understand the EXERCISE ADVICE above.
Signed   Date

Figure 10.2: **Exercise safety questionnaire.**

Techniques of Fitness Assessment

There are numerous methods available for assessing the various components of physical fitness. Some are elaborate and time-consuming, often requiring sophisticated equipment, but many others are simple, objective and reliable. Information from such assessments can provide information for a total fitness profile such as that shown in Table 10.18. The tests considered here in detail will cover the areas of anthropometry (body measurements), blood pressure, cardiovascular endurance, flexibility and muscular strength and endurance. Other sport-specific tests that assess agility, power, speed etc.

can be obtained from more detailed testing manuals. Table 10.1 shows some common tests used in the areas to be considered here.

Anthropometry

Measuring body fatness is a task frequently required of the Fitness Leader. The main anthropometric measures of value to the Fitness Leader are height, weight, girth and body composition. Height-to-weight ratios are also often used as a combined measure of obesity or overweight (i.e. the Ponderal or Quetelet indices). However, because these indices don't take into account the extent of lean body mass (LBM) and bony structure, they are usually inappropriate as a measure of fatness.

Fitness component	Tests	Comments
Cardiorespiratory endurance (VO₂ max)	Treadmill	Coupled with gas analysis, is the best test available.
	Bicycle ergometer	Simple yet accurate and safe.
	Bench stepping	Simple in design and operation.
	12 minute run	Field test with minimal facility.
Muscular strength and endurance	Sit-ups	Measures abdominal strength.
	Dynamometer	Measures handgrip strength, back lift and leg lift strength.
	Tensiometer	Measures strength of several muscle groups.
	Weight lifting	Measures absolute and relative strength and power.
Muscular endurance	Chin-ups	Measures arm, shoulder and back strength endurance.
	Flexed arm hang	Measures forearm, biceps, and upper back muscle endurance.
	Push-ups	Measures chest, shoulder and triceps muscular endurance.
	Sit-ups	Measures abdominal endurance.
Flexibility	Sit and reach test	Measures static flexibility at the hip joint.
	Leighton's flexometer	Measures flexibility of all joints in degrees.

Table 10.1: **Some common tests.**

It is important to note that in many cases the traditional measure of body weight is an invalid measure of changes in body composition. As a result of training, an individual can lose fat but gain LBM or muscle. Because muscle is heavier than fat, total body weight may increase rather than decrease in the early stages of training. Weight increases as a result of increases in lean tissue can counter weight losses in body fat, often leading to disillusionment of the client.

A more accurate guide to overfatness is the direct measurement of body fat. The original gold standard for this was underwater weighing, however more technologically advanced procedures like Magnetic Resonance Imagery (MRI) and Computerised Anthropometric Tomography (CAT scan) are now used to set standard standards for body fatness.

In most clinical or applied situations MRI and CAT scans are impractical and the next best method is the assessment of fat using skinfold measurements taken with special skinfold calipers.

General guide and comments

Taking accurate and repeatable skinfold measurements depends on accurate location of the sites of measurement.

The pointer on the dial of the skinfold caliper should be allowed to steady before measurements are recorded. Precise measuring and marking of the level of the skinfold are necessary because subcutaneous fat thickness varies substantially over the areas being measured.

Although skinfold measurements are generally simple to carry out, the correct procedure requires much practice. Tester error is the most common source of variation in measurements.

Common sites used (see Fig. 10.3)

Skinfold over the triceps: Located on the dorsum of the right upper arm (over the triceps), at the marked level halfway between the acromial process of the scapula and olecranon process (elbow). While measuring this skinfold, the arms should hang freely. The crest of the skinfold is parallel to the long axis of the upper arm.

Skinfold over biceps: Located on the ventral side of the upper arm (over the biceps), halfway between acromion and olecranon processes. The crest of the skinfold is parallel to the long axis of the upper arm.

Subscapular skin fold: Located about 1 cm below the lower angle of the right scapula with the subject standing in a relaxed position. The crest of the skinfold is medially upward and laterally downward at about 45°.

Suprailiac skin fold: Located about 3 cm above the suprailiac crest (hip bone). The crest of the skinfold is oblique with the natural line of the skin and muscle.

Chest skinfold: Located by plotting a mark along the lateral border of the pectoralis major, midway between the nipple and the anterior axillary fold of the armpit. The crest of the skinfold is oblique with the natural line of the skin and muscle.

Abdominal skinfold: Located 4cm laterally to right of the umbilicus and is taken vertically.

Mid-anterior thigh skinfold: Located by plotting a mark on the middle of the anterior aspect of the thigh midway between the anterior superior iliac spine and the superior aspect of the patella. The crest of the skinfold is vertical and parallel to the long axis of the femur.

British researchers Durnin and Womersley measured skinfold thickness at the triceps, biceps, suprailiac and subscapula sites and calibrated these with underwater weighing, deriving the equivalent fat content as a percentage of body weight. From this they developed generalised tables of body fat norms by age (see Table 10.2). Jackson and Pollock developed similar tables, but they provided for gender differences. Jackson and Pollock measured skinfold thickness of men at the chest, mid-abdominal and mid-anterior thigh, and women at the triceps, suprailiac and mid-anterior skinfolds (see Table 10.3).

Procedure

The skinfold caliper should have a pressure of 10 gm/mm, irrespective of the design of the caliper. A useful size of the contact surface is 20–40 mm and depends in part on the shape of the contact surface. The skin should be lifted by grasping a fold firmly between the thumb and forefinger at a distance of about 1 cm from the site at which the skinfold is to be measured.

1. With the crest of the fold following the alignment specified, apply the caliper jaws to the exact site, then release the spring handles fully.
2. When the pointer of the dial has steadied, read off the measurements in tenths of millimetres.
3. Take three readings at each site, allowing at least 15 seconds between measures, and take an average of the three readings.

Estimation of leanness and fatness

Using Tables 10.2 and 10.3 for Durnin and Womersley and Tables 10.4 and 10.5 for Jackson and Pollock, the sum of the averaged skinfolds can be converted to percent body fat. For example, if a sum total of the four skinfold thicknesses using the Durnin and Womersley protocol amounts to 74 mm, then using Tables 10.2 for men and 10.3 for women, one could read across the table on the column

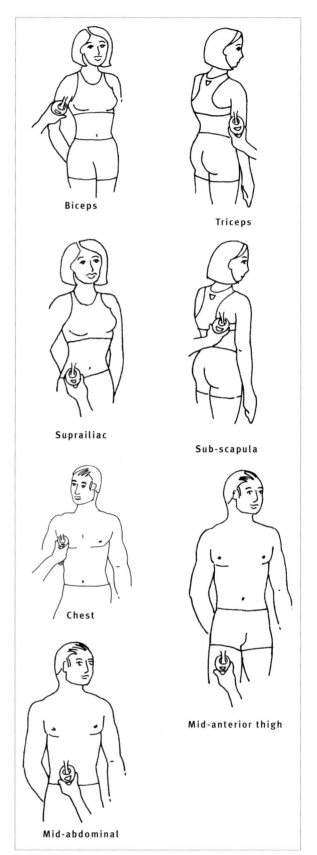

Figure 10.3: **Common skinfold sites.**

Sum of skinfolds (mm)	Males (age in years) 17–19	20–29	30–39	40–49	50+
15	5.00	4.64	9.09	8.47	8.38
16	5.75	5.58	9.74	9.31	9.31
17	6.44	6.08	10.35	10.09	10.19
18	7.10	6.74	10.93	10.84	11.02
19	7.72	7.37	11.48	11.54	11.80
20	8.32	7.96	12.00	12.22	12.55
21	8.89	8.53	12.50	12.86	13.27
22	9.43	9.07	12.97	13.47	13.95
23	9.95	9.59	13.43	14.06	14.60
24	10.45	10.09	13.87	14.62	15.23
25	10.92	10.57	14.29	15.16	15.84
26	11.39	11.03	14.69	15.68	16.42
27	11.83	11.48	15.08	16.19	16.98
28	12.26	11.91	15.46	16.67	17.53
29	12.67	12.32	15.82	17.14	18.05
30	13.07	12.73	16.17	17.60	18.56
31	13.46	13.12	16.51	18.04	19.05
32	13.84	13.49	16.84	18.47	19.53
33	14.21	13.86	17.16	18.88	19.99
34	14.56	14.22	17.47	19.28	20.44
35	14.91	14.56	17.77	19.68	20.88
36	15.25	14.90	18.07	20.06	21.31
37	15.57	15.23	18.36	20.43	21.73
38	15.89	15.55	18.63	20.79	22.13
39	16.21	15.86	18.91	21.15	22.53
40	16.51	16.17	19.17	21.49	22.92
41	16.81	16.47	19.43	21.83	23.29
42	17.10	16.76	19.69	22.16	23.66
43	17.38	17.04	19.93	22.48	24.02
44	17.66	17.32	20.18	22.80	24.38
45	17.93	17.59	20.41	23.11	24.72
46	18.20	17.86	20.65	23.41	25.06
47	18.46	18.12	20.87	23.71	25.39
48	18.71	18.37	21.10	24.00	25.72
49	18.96	18.63	21.31	24.28	26.04
50	19.21	18.87	21.53	24.56	26.35
51	19.45	19.11	21.74	24.83	26.66
52	19.69	19.35	21.95	25.10	26.96
53	19.92	19.58	22.15	25.37	27.26
54	20.15	19.81	22.35	25.63	27.55
55	20.37	20.04	22.54	25.88	27.83
56	20.59	20.26	22.73	26.13	28.11
57	20.81	20.47	22.92	26.38	28.39
58	21.02	20.69	23.11	26.62	28.66
59	21.23	20.90	23.29	26.86	28.93
60	21.44	21.11	23.47	27.09	29.20
61	21.64	21.31	23.65	27.33	29.45
62	21.84	21.51	23.82	27.55	29.71
63	22.04	21.71	23.99	27.78	29.96
64	22.23	21.90	24.16	28.00	30.21
65	22.42	22.09	24.33	28.22	30.45
66	22.61	22.28	24.49	28.43	30.70
67	22.80	22.47	24.66	28.64	30.93
68	22.98	22.65	24.81	28.85	31.17
69	23.16	22.83	24.97	29.06	31.40
70	23.34	23.01	25.13	29.26	31.63

Sum of skinfolds (mm)	Males (age in years) 17–19	20–29	30–39	40–49	50+
71	23.52	23.19	25.28	29.46	31.85
72	23.69	23.36	25.43	29.66	32.07
73	23.86	23.53	25.58	29.85	32.29
74	24.03	23.70	25.73	30.04	32.51
75	24.20	23.87	25.87	30.23	32.72
76	24.36	24.03	26.01	30.42	32.93
77	24.52	24.20	26.16	30.61	33.14
78	24.68	24.36	26.30	30.79	33.35
79	24.84	24.52	26.43	30.97	33.55
80	25.00	24.67	26.57	31.15	33.75
81	25.15	24.83	26.70	31.33	33.95
82	25.31	24.98	26.84	31.50	34.15
83	25.46	25.13	26.97	31.67	34.34
84	25.61	25.28	27.10	31.85	34.53
85	25.76	25.43	27.23	32.01	34.72
86	25.90	25.58	27.36	32.18	34.91
87	26.05	25.72	27.48	32.35	35.10
88	26.19	25.87	27.61	32.51	35.28
89	26.33	26.01	27.73	32.67	35.46
90	26.47	26.15	27.85	32.83	35.64
91	26.61	26.29	27.97	32.99	35.82
92	26.75	26.42	28.09	33.15	36.00
93	26.89	26.56	28.21	33.30	36.17
94	27.02	26.70	28.32	33.45	36.35
95	27.15	26.83	28.44	33.61	36.52
96	27.28	26.96	28.55	33.76	36.69
97	27.42	27.09	28.67	33.91	36.85
98	27.54	27.22	28.78	34.05	37.02
99	27.67	27.35	28.89	34.20	37.19
100	27.80	27.48	29.00	34.34	37.35
101	27.92	27.60	29.11	34.49	37.51
102	28.05	27.73	29.22	34.63	37.67
103	28.17	27.85	29.33	34.77	37.83
104	28.29	27.97	29.43	34.91	37.99
105	28.42	28.09	29.54	35.05	38.14
106	28.54	28.21	29.64	35.19	38.30
107	28.65	28.33	29.74	35.32	38.45
108	28.77	28.45	29.85	35.46	38.60
109	28.89	28.57	29.95	35.59	38.75
110	29.00	28.68	30.05	35.72	38.90
111	29.12	28.80	30.15	35.85	39.05
112	29.23	28.91	30.25	35.98	39.20
113	29.35	29.03	30.34	36.11	39.34
114	29.46	29.14	30.44	36.24	39.48
115	29.57	29.25	30.54	36.37	39.63
116	29.68	29.36	30.63	36.49	39.77
117	29.79	29.47	30.73	36.62	39.91
118	29.90	29.58	30.82	36.74	40.05
119	30.00	29.69	30.91	36.86	40.19
120	30.11	29.79	31.01	36.99	40.33
121	30.22	29.90	31.10	37.11	40.46
122	30.32	30.00	31.19	37.23	40.60
123	30.43	30.11	31.28	37.35	40.73
124	30.53	30.21	31.37	37.46	40.87
125	30.63	30.31	31.46	37.58	41.00

Table 10.2: **Percent body fat by age — males. (Durnin and Womersley, 1974)**

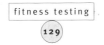

Sum of skinfolds mm	Females (age in years) 17-19	20–29	30–39	40–49	50+
15	10.40	10.22	13.50	16.40	17.85
16	11.21	11.08	14.27	17.15	18.65
17	11.98	11.89	14.99	17.87	19.40
18	12.71	12.66	15.68	18.54	20.11
19	13.40	13.39	16.33	19.18	20.79
20	14.05	14.08	16.95	19.78	21.44
21	14.68	14.75	17.54	20.36	22.05
22	15.28	15.38	18.10	20.92	22.64
23	15.85	15.99	18.64	21.45	23.20
24	16.40	16.57	19.16	21.96	23.74
25	16.93	17.13	19.66	22.44	24.26
26	17.44	17.67	20.14	22.91	24.76
27	17.93	18.19	20.60	23.37	25.24
28	18.40	18.69	21.05	23.80	25.71
29	18.86	19.17	21.48	24.23	26.16
30	19.30	19.64	21.90	24.64	26.59
31	19.73	20.10	22.31	25.03	27.01
32	20.15	20.54	22.70	25.42	27.42
33	20.56	20.97	23.08	25.79	27.82
34	20.95	21.39	23.45	26.16	28.21
35	21.33	21.79	23.81	26.51	28.58
36	21.71	22.19	24.16	26.85	28.95
37	22.07	22.57	24.51	27.19	29.30
38	22.42	22.95	24.84	27.51	29.65
39	22.77	23.31	25.16	27.83	29.99
40	23.10	23.67	25.48	28.14	30.32
41	23.43	24.02	25.79	28.45	30.64
42	23.76	24.36	26.09	28.74	30.96
43	24.07	24.69	26.39	29.03	31.26
44	24.38	25.02	26.68	29.32	31.57
45	24.68	25.34	26.96	29.59	31.86
46	24.97	25.65	27.24	29.87	32.15
47	25.26	25.96	27.51	30.13	32.43
48	25.54	26.26	27.78	30.39	32.71
49	25.82	26.55	28.04	30.65	32.98
50	26.09	26.84	28.30	30.90	33.25
51	26.36	27.12	28.55	31.14	33.51
52	26.62	27.40	28.79	31.39	33.77
53	26.88	27.68	29.04	31.62	34.02
54	27.13	27.94	29.27	31.86	34.27
55	27.38	28.21	29.51	32.09	34.51
56	27.63	28.47	29.74	32.31	34.75
57	27.87	28.72	29.96	32.53	34.99
58	28.10	28.97	30.19	32.75	35.22
59	28.34	29.22	30.40	32.96	35.45
60	28.57	29.46	30.62	33.17	35.67
61	28.79	29.70	30.83	33.38	35.89
62	29.01	29.94	31.04	33.58	36.11
63	29.23	30.17	31.25	33.79	36.32
64	29.45	30.40	31.45	33.98	36.53
65	29.66	30.62	31.65	34.18	36.74
66	29.87	30.84	31.84	34.37	36.95
67	30.07	31.06	32.04	34.56	37.15
68	30.28	31.28	32.23	34.74	37.35
69	30.48	31.49	32.32	34.93	37.54
70	30.67	31.70	32.60	35.11	37.74

Sum of skinfolds mm	Females (age in years) 17-19	20–29	30–39	40–49	50+
71	30.87	31.91	32.79	35.29	37.93
72	31.06	32.11	32.97	35.47	38.12
73	31.25	32.32	33.14	35.64	38.30
74	31.44	32.51	33.32	35.82	38.49
75	31.62	32.71	33.49	35.99	38.67
76	31.81	32.91	33.67	36.15	38.85
77	31.99	33.10	33.84	36.32	39.02
78	32.17	33.29	34.00	36.48	39.20
79	32.34	33.47	34.17	36.65	29.37
80	32.52	33.66	34.33	36.81	39.54
81	32.69	33.84	34.49	36.96	39.71
82	32.86	34.02	34.65	37.12	39.88
83	33.03	34.20	34.81	37.28	40.04
84	33.19	34.38	34.97	37.43	40.20
85	33.36	34.55	35.12	37.58	40.36
86	33.52	34.73	35.28	37.73	40.52
87	33.68	34.90	35.43	37.88	40.68
88	33.84	35.07	35.58	38.02	40.84
89	34.00	35.23	35.72	38.17	40.99
90	34.15	35.40	35.87	38.31	41.14
91	34.31	35.56	36.01	38.45	41.29
92	34.46	35.72	36.16	38.59	41.44
93	34.61	35.88	36.30	38.73	41.59
94	34.76	36.04	36.44	38.87	41.74
95	34.91	36.20	36.58	39.00	41.88
96	35.06	36.36	36.72	39.14	42.03
97	35.20	36.51	36.85	39.27	42.17
98	35.34	36.66	36.99	39.40	42.31
99	35.49	36.82	37.12	39.53	42.45
100	35.63	36.97	37.25	39.66	42.59
101	35.77	37.11	37.38	39.79	42.72
102	35.91	37.26	37.51	39.92	42.86
103	36.04	37.41	37.64	40.04	42.99
104	36.18	37.55	37.77	40.17	43.13
105	36.31	37.69	37.90	40.29	43.26
106	36.45	37.84	38.02	40.41	43.39
107	36.58	37.98	38.15	40.54	43.52
108	36.71	38.12	38.27	40.66	43.65
109	36.84	38.25	38.39	40.77	43.77
110	36.97	38.39	38.51	40.89	43.90
111	37.10	38.53	38.63	41.01	44.02
112	37.22	38.66	38.75	41.13	44.15
113	37.35	38.80	38.87	41.24	44.27
114	37.47	38.93	38.98	41.36	44.39
115	37.60	39.06	39.10	41.47	44.51
116	37.72	39.19	39.21	41.58	44.63
117	37.84	39.32	39.33	41.69	44.75
118	37.96	39.45	39.44	41.80	44.87
119	38.08	39.57	39.55	41.91	44.99
120	38.20	39.70	39.66	42.02	45.10
121	38.32	39.83	39.78	42.13	45.22
122	38.43	39.95	39.88	42.24	45.33
123	38.55	40.07	39.99	42.34	45.45
124	38.66	40.20	40.10	42.45	45.56
125	38.78	40.32	40.21	42.55	45.67

Table 10.3: **Percent body fat by age — females. (Durnin and Womersley, 1974)**

Sum of skinfolds	Percent fat estimate for women: Sum of triceps, suprailiac, and thigh skinfolds								
	under 22	23–27	28–32	33–37	38–42	43–47	48–52	53–57	over 57
23–25	9.7	9.9	10.2	10.4	10.7	10.9	11.2	11.4	11.7
26–28	11.0	11.2	11.5	11.7	12.0	12.3	12.5	12.7	13.0
29–31	12.3	12.5	12.8	13.0	13.3	13.5	13.8	14.0	14.3
32–34	13.6	13.8	14.0	14.3	14.5	14.8	15.0	15.3	15.5
35–37	14.8	15.0	15.3	15.5	15.8	16.0	16.3	16.5	16.8
38–40	16.0	16.3	16.5	16.7	17.0	`17.2	17.5	17.7	18.0
41–43	17.2	17.4	17.7	17.9	18.2	18.4	18.7	18.9	19.2
44–46	18.3	18.6	18.8	19.1	19.3	19.6	19.8	20.1	20.3
47–49	19.5	19.7	20.0	20.2	20.5	20.7	21.0	21.2	21.5
50–52	20.6	20.8	21.1	21.3	21.6	21.8	22.1	22.3	22.6
53–55	21.7	21.9	22.1	22.4	22.6	22.9	23.1	23.4	23.6
56–58	22.7	23.0	23.2	23.4	23.7	23.9	24.2	24.4	24.7
59–61	23.7	24.0	24.2	24.5	24.7	25.0	25.2	25.5	25.7
62–64	24.7	25.0	25.2	25.5	25.7	26.0	26.2	26.4	26.7
65–67	25.7	25.9	26.2	26.4	26.7	26.9	27.2	27.4	27.7
68–70	26.6	26.9	27.1	27.4	27.6	27.9	28.1	28.4	28.6
71–73	27.5	27.8	28.0	28.3	28.5	28.8	29.0	29.3	29.5
74–76	28.4	28.7	28.9	29.2	29.4	29.7	29.9	30.2	30.4
77–79	29.3	29.5	29.8	30.0	30.3	30.5	30.8	31.0	31.3
80–82	30.1	30.4	30.6	30.9	21.1	31.4	31.6	31.9	32.1
83–85	30.9	31.2	31.4	31.7	31.9	32.2	32.4	32.7	32.9
86–88	31.7	32.0	32.3	32.5	32.7	32.9	33.2	33.4	33.7
89–91	32.5	32.7	33.0	33.2	33.5	33.7	33.9	34.2	34.4
92–94	33.2	33.4	33.7	33.9	34.2	34.4	34.7	34.9	35.2
95–97	33.9	34.1	34.4	34.6	34.9	35.1	35.4	35.6	35.9
98–100	34.6	34.8	35.1	35.3	35.5	35.8	36.0	36.3	36.5
101–103	35.3	35.4	35.7	35.9	36.2	36.4	36.7	36.9	37.2
104–106	35.8	36.1	36.3	36.6	36.8	37.1	37.3	37.5	37.8
107–109	36.4	36.7	36.9	37.1	37.4	37.6	37.9	38.1	38.4
110–112	37.0	37.2	37.5	37.7	38.0	38.2	38.5	38.7	38.9
113–115	37.5	37.8	38.0	38.2	38.5	38.7	39.0	39.2	39.5
116–118	38.0	38.3	38.5	38.8	39.0	39.3	39.5	39.7	40.0
119–121	38.5	38.7	39.0	39.2	39.5	39.7	40.0	40.2	40.5
122–124	39.0	39.2	39.4	39.7	39.9	40.2	40.4	40.7	40.9
125–127	39.4	39.6	39.9	40.1	40.4	40.6	40.9	41.1	41.4
128–130	39.8	40.0	40.3	40.5	40.8	41.0	41.3	41.5	41.8

Table 10.4: **Percent fat estimate by age — women. (Jackson & Pollock, 1985)**

with the appropriate age group. For a man aged 35 years with a skinfold thickness of 74 mm, his percent body fat is 25.73. This means that 25.7% of his body weight is made up of fat tissue, i.e. 18 kg of adipose tissue is present in his body if his body weight is 70 kg. The corresponding value for a woman is 33.32% or 20 kg of fat in a body weighing 60 kg.

The average fat content for a young, healthy adult man is 10–15% and for a young, healthy adult woman is 18–25%. On average, older men and women have approximately 5–10% more fat than their younger counterparts. However, the increase in body fat content with age is not necessarily physiologically desirable or healthy. Classification of leanness and fatness based on

percent body fat is necessarily arbitrary. Nevertheless, Table 10.6 gives an arbitrary classification for the general population.

Body fat content is obviously affected by physical activity. There is a wide variation in body fat content ranging from 4–20% for male athletes, and 10–26% for female athletes. Certainly the types of sporting activity and the amount of physical training involved are important determinants of body composition in elite athletes. Again, classification of leanness and fatness for average athletes is necessarily arbitrary. Table 10.7 serves as a guide for such a classification.

When taking skinfold measures and counselling people on their percent body fat levels, instructors

Sum of Skinfolds(mm)	Percent fat estimate for males: sum of chest, abdomen, and thigh skinfolds							
⋯ 22	23–27	28–32	33–37	38–42	43–47	48–52	53–57	over 57
8–10	1.3	1.8	2.3	2.9	3.4	3.9	4.5	5.0	5.5
11–13	2.2	2.8	3.3	3.9	4.4	4.9	5.5	6.0	6.5
14–16	3.2	3.8	4.3	4.8	5.4	5.9	6.4	7.0	7.5
17–19	4.2	4.7	5.3	5.8	6.3	6.9	7.4	8.0	8.5
20–22	5.1	5.7	6.2	6.8	7.3	7.9	8.4	8.9	9.5
23–25	9.7	9.9	10.2	10.4	10.7	10.9	11.2	11.4	11.7
26–28	11.0	11.2	11.5	11.7	12.0	12.3	12.5	12.7	13.0
29–31	12.3	12.5	12.8	13.0	13.3	13.5	13.8	14.0	14.3
32–34	13.6	13.8	14.0	14.3	14.5	14.8	15.0	15.3	15.5
35–37	14.8	15.0	15.3	15.5	15.8	16.0	16.3	16.5	16.8
38–40	16.0	16.3	16.5	16.7	17.0	`17.2	17.5	17.7	18.0
41–43	17.2	17.4	17.7	17.9	18.2	18.4	18.7	18.9	19.2
44–46	18.3	18.6	18.8	19.1	19.3	19.6	19.8	20.1	20.3
47–49	19.5	19.7	20.0	20.2	20.5	20.7	21.0	21.2	21.5
50–52	20.6	20.8	21.1	21.3	21.6	21.8	22.1	22.3	22.6
53–55	21.7	21.9	22.1	22.4	22.6	22.9	23.1	23.4	23.6
56–58	22.7	23.0	23.2	23.4	23.7	23.9	24.2	24.4	24.7
59–61	23.7	24.0	24.2	24.5	24.7	25.0	25.2	25.5	25.7
62–64	24.7	25.0	25.2	25.5	25.7	26.0	26.2	26.4	26.7
65–67	25.7	25.9	26.2	26.4	26.7	26.9	27.2	27.4	27.7
68–70	26.6	26.9	27.1	27.4	27.6	27.9	28.1	28.4	28.6
71–73	27.5	27.8	28.0	28.3	28.5	28.8	29.0	29.3	29.5
74–76	28.4	28.7	28.9	29.2	29.4	29.7	29.9	30.2	30.4
77–79	29.3	29.5	29.8	30.0	30.3	30.5	30.8	31.0	31.3
80–82	30.1	30.4	30.6	30.9	21.1	31.4	31.6	31.9	32.1
83–85	30.9	31.2	31.4	31.7	31.9	32.2	32.4	32.7	32.9
86–88	31.7	32.0	32.3	32.5	32.7	32.9	33.2	33.4	33.7
89–91	32.5	32.7	33.0	33.2	33.5	33.7	33.9	34.2	34.4
92–94	33.2	33.4	33.7	33.9	34.2	34.4	34.7	34.9	35.2
95–97	33.9	34.1	34.4	34.6	34.9	35.1	35.4	35.6	35.9
98–100	34.6	34.8	35.1	35.3	35.5	35.8	36.0	36.3	36.5
101–103	35.3	35.4	35.7	35.9	36.2	36.4	36.7	36.9	37.2
104–106	35.8	36.1	36.3	36.6	36.8	37.1	37.3	37.5	37.8
107–109	36.4	36.7	36.9	37.1	37.4	37.6	37.9	38.1	38.4
110–112	37.0	37.2	37.5	37.7	38.0	38.2	38.5	38.7	38.9
113–115	37.5	37.8	38.0	38.2	38.5	38.7	39.0	39.2	39.5
116–118	38.0	38.3	38.5	38.8	39.0	39.3	39.5	39.7	40.0
119–121	38.5	38.7	39.0	39.2	39.5	39.7	40.0	40.2	40.5
122–124	39.0	39.2	39.4	39.7	39.9	40.2	40.4	40.7	40.9
125–127	39.4	39.6	39.9	40.1	40.4	40.6	40.9	41.1	41.4

Table 10.5: **Percent body fat by age — men. (Jackson and Pollock, 1985)**

should be sensitive to the feelings of the client. Terms such as 'moderately obese' and 'body fat' should be replaced with 'higher than average' and 'extra weight'.

Girth measurements

Girth measurements are a useful method of evaluating changes in body shape. As fat stores are reduced, fat cells shrink and as a result the circumference of body segments decreases. They are a useful substitute for skinfold measures where the client is extremely overweight.

Girth measurements are taken in the transverse plane; common sites are:

Chest: at the nipple line during the mid point of a normal breath.

Waist: at the narrowest point, below the rib cage and above the hip bones (females only), and males at the umbilicus.

Hips: with the feet together, at the level of the symphysis pubis in front and at the maximal protrusion of the buttocks at the back.

	Men	Women
Lean	←····12.0%	←····17%
Acceptable	12–20.9%	17–27.0%
Mod. overweight	21–25.9%	28–32.9%
Overweight	····⟩ 26%	····⟩ 33%

Table 10.6: **Classification of leanness and fatness based on percent body fat for general population.**

	Male athletes	Female athletes
Lean	←····7.0%	←····12.0%
Acceptable	7–14%	12–24.9%
Overweight	····⟩ 15.0%	····⟩ 25.0%

Table 10.7: **Classification of leanness and fatness for male and female athletes based on percent body fat.**

Thigh: at the crotch level and just below the fold of the buttocks.

Calf: at the maximal circumference.

Upper arm: at the maximal circumference; arm extended, palm up.

Remember that there are no 'norms' for girth measurements; they are used primarily for documenting changes that may be occurring in different body areas due to your client's change in lifestyle.

Waist-to-hip ratio (WHR)

WHR is an objective means of measuring body fat distribution above and below the waist. It is calculated simply by dividing an individual's girth at the waist (a level measure at the umbilicus) by their hip girth (taken at the widest point from a lateral view). This method of measurement differentiates between the android (apple) shape characterised by males and the gynoid (pear) shape characterised by women. Men and women with a WHR > 0.9 and > 0.8 respectively are considered to be at greater risk of ill health.

Blood Pressure

Blood pressure is the measure of the force the heart needs to push blood through the body. A simple definition of blood pressure is: 'The resistance of the blood against the artery walls'.

A good analogy, when explaining blood pressure, is the force of water in a hose pipe. If the hose is thin or blocked in any way, the same force of water at the tap will cause a higher pressure against the walls of the hose. If, on the other hand, the hose has a large opening and the water is free flowing, the pressure of the water against the hose will be low. The same is true for the arterial blood vessels. If there is too much pressure on the artery walls this places additional strain on the heart.

There are two different measures of blood pressure:
The systolic measure: which is the contraction phase of the heart or the pumping pressure of the heart
The diastolic measure: which is the relaxation phase of the heart or the pressure in the arteries when the heart is filling up with blood.

These two measures are expressed as systolic over diastolic and an acceptable range is considered to be:

Systolic 120 ± 10
Diastolic 80 ± 10

Recording blood pressure

Blood pressures can be measured by the auscultatory method, using a sphygmomanometer and a stethoscope. A sphygmomanometer consists of a cuff, a mercury manometer (or anaroid manometer), and an inflating bulb with exhaust control (see Fig. 10.4). The stethoscope is used to listen to the sounds of blood flow. The cuff is wrapped around the arm. When the brachial artery is occluded by increasing the cuff pressure 30 mm Hg above the expected systolic pressure, there is no blood flowing to the forearm and no sound is heard through the stethoscope. As the cuff pressure is lowered slowly to a point at which systolic blood pressure just exceeds the cuff pressure, a tapping sound can be heard. The cuff pressure at which the first sound is heard is called the systolic blood pressure. As the cuff pressure is lowered further, the sound becomes louder, then dull and muffled, and finally disappears. These are the 'sounds of Korotkow'. The abrupt muffling of the arterial sound signals that blood flow is no longer impeded by the cuff pressure, and this is the diastolic blood pressure.

Blood pressures are usually expressed in millimetres of mercury (mmHg).

Instructors are reminded that anyone can take blood pressure, but diagnosis and counselling of hypertension should be done only by appropriately medically qualified people.

Blood pressures vary considerably throughout the day and night, according to a variety of conditions. Posture, breathing, emotion, exercise, cigarette smoking and caffeine can cause a rise or fall in blood pressure. If a subject has not engaged in physical activity for 2 hours prior to testing, has not been under emotional stress, has not been smoking or drinking caffeinated beverages for the previous 2 hours and has been seated comfortably for half an hour prior to blood pressure recording, variations can be minimised and false diagnoses can be avoided.

The World Health Organization has defined a systolic blood pressure of more than 160 mmHg and a diastolic blood pressure of more than 95 mmHg as abnormal and requiring treatment and continuous observation. Blood pressure consistently below 140 mmHg for systolic and 90 mmHg for diastolic can be regarded as being normal.

The National Heart Foundation states that a person who records a blood pressure measure of 140/90 has borderline hypertension (high blood pressure) and further medical examination is recommended. This is especially recommended if the person wishes to participate in an exercise program.

Procedure

1. Sit the subject with arm outstretched. Loosen the control valve on the cuff of the 'sphygmo' by turning it anti-clockwise so that air is released entirely from the cuff.
2. Wrap the cuff around the subject's arm, with the lower edge 2 cm above the crease at the elbow. Ensure that the stethoscope on the cuff is against the skin.
3. Close the control valve and pump the bulb to raise the cuff pressure to a level of about 160–180 mmHg on the manometer.
4. Gradually open the control valve so that the needle slowly moves downward as the cuff pressure is released. The rate of pressure drop should be 2–3 mmHg per second.

5. The first sound heard through the stethoscope indicates the pressure at which blood again begins to flow to the forearm. This is taken as the systolic blood pressure.
6. Allow the cuff pressure to continue to fall. Note that the sound becomes louder, then dull and muffled, and disappears altogether. The point at which the sound becomes muffled is the diastolic blood pressure.
7. Deflate the cuff entirely. Allow for 1–2 minutes rest and repeat the above procedure to obtain a second reading.

Evaluating Cardiorespiratory Endurance (Stamina)

Cardiorespiratory endurance can be measured in a number of ways, the standard being the direct measurement of oxygen uptake. This requires sophisticated equipment to measure expired respiratory gases while the subject is exercising at a maximal level. Measurements can be carried out on a treadmill, exercise bicycle, rowing machine or similar aerobic exercise machine.

For practicality, the maximum (or 'max') test is not always appropriate but a number of sub-maximal tests can be used. In these cases, the subject is exercised to a pre-set level (not exhaustion), and extrapolations are made from norm tables to estimate maximal oxygen uptake (VO_2 max).

Submaximal aerobic tests estimate maximal oxygen uptake (VO_2 max) based on heart rate following a set workload. This estimate is based on the physiological principle that there is a direct and linear relationship between heart rate and workload (see Fig. 10.4).

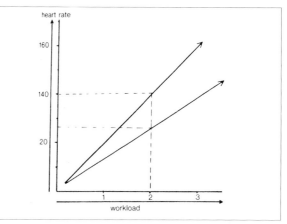

Figure 10.4: **Relationship between heart rate and workload.**

Test	Time required	Procedure	Advantages	Disadvantages	Estimated relation with VO2 max test
12–15 min. run	12–15 mins	Distance covered; formulae for determining VO2 for trained and untrained athletes	• Simplicity • No equipment	• Needs practice for pacing • Favours runners/walkers • High stress leveL	85–90%
Astrand bicycle ergometer	6 mins	Constant workload on cycle ergometer, VO2 max estimated from tables of heart rate (HR). HR taken between 5th & 6th minute	• Time • Simplicity • Reasonably appropriate for ECG monitoring	• Variability in Max HR in individuals • Favours cyclists • Underestimates for those with a high maximum HR • As max HR decreases with age, the test over-estimates fitness with advancing age.	89–90%
PWC170	9 mins	3 workloads on cycle ergometer at 3 min intervals. By graphing HR responses to these workloads, work which can be completed at a HR of 170 can be estimated	• Clear steps on protocol • Gradual increase in work intensity • Reasonably accurate • Appropriate for ECG monitoring	• Time involved in graphing results • Difficulty in gauging 170 bpm level accurately • Favours cyclists	89–90%
Harvard Step Test	3–5 mins + 3 mins measuring	Step at rate of 30 steps/ min on 45.5 cm step. HR recorded at 1½, 2½ and 3½ mins. after stopping	• Minimal equipment • Easy to conduct • Can be self administering	• High stress level • Inappropriate for children • Influenced by variations in max HR	60–80%
Queen's College Step Test	3 mins + 15 secs. measuring	Step at rate of 24 steps/min (men), 22 steps/min (women) on 42.5 cm step. HR recorded for 15 secs, 5 secs after stopping.	• Minimal equipment • Easy to conduct • Little time required • Can be self administering	• Influenced by variations in max HR	

Table 10.8: **Advantages and disadvantages of common sub-maximal VO2 max tests.**

As aerobic fitness improves there is a reduction in heart rate for the same workload (Fig. 10.4). This is the basis of all submaximal tests that use heart rate as a measure of intensity. It should be noted, however, that the heart rate and workload relationships are only valid at a certain heart rate range and are not linear at very high or very low heart rates. Thus, given a certain workload, and the heart rate measured at the steady state of work the maximum oxygen uptake can be predicted with a known degree of accuracy.

The advantages and disadvantages of the most common submaximal tests are summarised in Table 10.8.

A Sub-maximal Test Using the Bicycle Ergometer

Although VO$_2$ max is primarily dependent on the cardiorespiratory function of man, it is also related to the duration and nature of the task, the mass of muscle involved, fatigue levels, and environmental conditions such as climate and altitude.

The bicycle ergometer is perhaps the most adaptable instrument in the laboratory for aerobic testing. It is simple to use, cheap, occupies little space and is easily transportable. It's also sufficiently versatile to assume a number of different work loads.

Work on the bicycle ergometer is calculated in kilopondmetres/minute. A kilopondmetre (kpm) is the amount of force required to move a mass of 1 kg through a distance of 1 metre. A watt (which is also often used as a measure of work) equals 6.12 kpm/min.

Before being tested on the bicycle ergometer, a subject should satisfy the following:

Pre-testing conditions

1. No meal should be taken for 1–2 hours prior to the test.
2. No vigorous exercise for at least 24 hours.
3. No smoking for 1 hour.
4. No caffeinated drinks (tea, coffee, cola) for at least 1 hour.

5. Subjects on blood pressure medication should consult their doctor about refraining from medication for 24 hours prior to testing, if possible.

Testing procedure

The following is the testing procedure for an Astrand/Rhyming sub-maximal bicycle test.

1. Testing should be carried out in an environment of approximately 20^0 C.
2. Ensure the subject is comfortable on the bike. Saddle height should allow for completely stretched leg at the lowest pedal point.
3. Practise taking resting pulse while the subject is seated. This can be done at either the neck (carotid pulse) or wrist (radial pulse). If a heart rate meter or electrocardiograph (ECG) is used, these should be regularly calibrated.
4. Determine a workload suitable for the subject.
5. After commencing exercise, ensure that the subject is pedalling at a steady pace at the desired workload. While pedalling, the subject should remain seated.
6. After 1 minute of exercise, a satisfactory heart rate would be 116–128 bpm. An underload or overload would be noticed at 1–2 minutes and appropriate adjustments made to the work load.
7. The ideal heart rate of steady state of exercise is 120–170 beats per minute (depending on age).
8. Measure heart rate for 15 seconds every minute on the minute and multiply this by 4 to get HR per minute. This should be done for 7 minutes and scores recorded on a data sheet.
9. Average the 5th and 6th minutes of heart rate if there was no alteration of work load since the start of exercise; otherwise average the 6th and 7th minutes of heart rates. Enter this average heart rate as the work heart rate.
10. Record the workload at this point on the data sheet.
11. If the subject experiences discomfort while exercising, the test should be stopped immediately.

Calculation of VO₂ max

Using the working heart rate and the exercise load, VO₂ max can be calculated from the tables provided for men and women (Tables 10.9 and 10.10).

As maximum heart rate decreases with age, a correction factor for age is needed. This can be done by multiplying the maximum oxygen uptake with the correction factor for the appropriate age range (see Table 10.11).

The figures provided by the following tables are in litres per minute. This can be converted to millilitres per minute by multiplying by 1000. A measure for VO₂ max can then be determined by dividing by body weight (in kilograms).

Example of a VO₂ max calculation

Age:	35 years
Sex:	Male
Body weight:	72.0 kg
Workload:	900 kpm/min
Heart rate:	147 bpm
Predicted VO₂ max:	3.3 litres/min (Table 10.9)
Age correction factor:	3.3 l/min x 0.87 (Table 10.11) = 2.871 l/min
VO₂ max expressed on a weight basis:	2.871 x 1000/72.0 = 39.8 ml/kg/min
Comparison tables:	Average VO₂ max for age

Standards for VO₂ max

Australian standards for maximum oxygen uptake are scarce, although tables have been developed from work carried out by the Human Performance Laboratory at the Sydney College of Advanced Education. Table 10.12 gives fitness levels for men and women aged 20–59. Table 10.13 gives comparative figures for Australian boys and girls.

A less accurate but more convenient sub-maximal measure of aerobic capacity for the fitness centre is the step test. There are a number of different step test measures, the two most common being the Harvard Step Test and the Queen's College Step Test.

Step Tests

The Harvard Step Test

The Harvard Step Test is based on heart rate recovery following a given work load. This consists of 3 or 5 minutes of stepping up and down on an 46 cm step, followed by pulse measurements at the first, second and third minutes after finishing stepping.

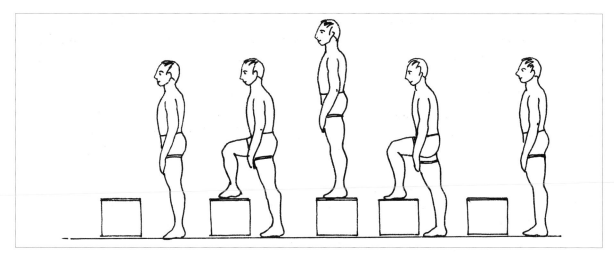

Figure 10.5: **Measuring aerobic fitness using the step test.**

The Queen's College Step Test

The Queen's College is a simpler step test developed by Professor William McArdle. This test is based on heart rate following a given workload, not recovery heart rate as is the case with the Harvard Step Test.

Testing procedure for the Queen's College Step Test:

1. Use a 41 cm step and have a cadence tape or metronome to ensure the correct stepping speed.
2. Have the subject start with both feet on the floor and facing the step. Practice the stepping cycle as follows:

   up — right foot up
   up — left foot up
   down — right foot down
   down — left foot down

Ensure that when on the step both legs are straight (see Fig. 10.5).

3. Once the subject has started stepping he or she must keep in time with the cadence. For women this should be 22 stepping cycles per minute and for men 24 stepping cycles.
4. The subject must maintain the stepping cycle for three minutes. However, after 1½ minutes the subject changes the leg he or she started stepping up on. This prevents too much overload on one leg.
5. Throughout the test the instructor should regularly monitor how the subject is feeling. If the subject feels any discomfort the test should be stopped and the heart rate and duration of the test recorded.
6. Immediately following 3 minutes of stepping the subject should stop and sit on the step. Within five seconds the instructor should begin counting heart rate for 15 seconds. Multiply this by 4 to give the heart rate per minute.
7. Compare the result with the scores from Table 10.14.

Estimates have also been made of VO_2 max from step tests, but it should be emphasised that, like all sub-maximal tests, these are subject to error.

Evaluating Flexibility

Flexibility is the ability to move part or parts of the body in a wide range of movement without undue strain to the articulations and muscle attachments. Since the range of movement in various joints of the same individual may differ greatly, flexibility is considered specific to the joint involved. By the proper use of standard instruments and tests it is possible to determine which individuals (and which joints of the body) have the greatest flexibility.

For many sports, flexibility is all-important. In the normal person, graceful movement in walking and running is dependent on a certain amount of flexibility. It is also believed that maintaining good joint mobility can prevent or relieve the aches and pains that grow more common with age.

Males Maximum Oxygen Uptake Litres/min.				
Heart Rate	kpm/min.	kpm/min.	kpm/min.	kpm/min.	kpm/min.
300	600	900	1200	1500	
120	2.2	3.5	4.8		
121	2.2	3.4	4.7		
122	2.2	3.4	4.6		
123	2.1	3.4	4.6		
124	2.1	3.3	4.5	6.0	
125	2.0	3.2	4.4	5.9	
126	2.0	3.2	4.4	5.8	
127	2.0	3.1	4.3	5.7	
128	2.0	3.1	4.2	5.6	
129	1.9	3.0	4.2	5.6	
130	1.9	3.0	4.1	5.5	
131	1.9	2.9	4.0	5.4	
132	1.8	2.9	4.0	5.3	
133	1.8	2.8	3.9	5.3	
134	1.8	2.8	3.9	5.2	
135	1.7	2.8	3.8	5.1	
136	1.7	2.7	3.8	5.0	
137	1.7	2.7	3.7	5.0	
138	1.6	2.7	3.7	4.9	
139	1.6	2.6	3.6	4.8	
140	1.6	2.6	3.6	4.8	6.0
141		2,6	3.5	4.7	5.9
142		2.5	3.5	4.6	5.8
143		2.5	3.4	4.6	5.7
144		2.5	3.4	4.5	5.7
145		2.4	3.4	4.5	5.6
146		2.4	3.3	4.4	5.6
147		2.4	3.3	4.4	5.5
148		2.4	3.2	4.3	5.4
149		2.3	3.2	4.3	5.4
150		2.3	3.2	4.2	5.3
151		2.3	3.1	4.2	5.2
152		2.3	3.1	4.1	5.2
153		2.2	3.0	4.1	5.1
154		2.2	3.0	4.0	5.1
155		2.2	3.0	4.0	5.0
156		2.2	2,9	4.0	5.0
157		2.1	2.9	3,9	4.9
158		2.1	2.9	3.9	4.9
159		2.1	2.8	3.8	4.8
160		2.1	2.8	3.8	4.8
161		2.0	2.8	3.7	4,7
162		2.0	2.8	3.7	4.6
163		2.0	2.8	3.7	4.6
164		2.0	2.7	3.6	4.5
165		2.0	2.7	3.6	4.5
166		1.9	2.7	3.6	4.5
167		1.9	2,6	3.5	4.4
168		1.9	2.6	3.5	4.4
169		1.9	2.6	3.5	4.3
170		1.8	2.6	3.4	4.3

Table 10.9: **Prediction of maximum oxygen uptake (males) from heart rate and work load on a bicycle ergometer.**

Females Maximum Oxygen Uptake Litres/min.				
Heart Rate	kpm/min.	kpm/min.	kpm/min.	kpm/min.	kpm/min.
300	450	600	750	900	
120	2.6	3.4	4.1	4.8	
121	2.5	3.3	4.0	4.8	
122	2.5	3.2	3.9	4.7	
123	2.4	3.1	3.9	4.6	
124	2.4	3.1	3.8	4.5	
125	2.3	3.0	3.7	4.4	
126	2.3	3.0	3.6	4.3	
127	2.2	2.9	3.5	4.2	
128	2.2	2.8	3.5	4.2	4.8
129	2.2	2.8	3.4	4.1	4.8
130	2.1	2.7	3.4	4.0	4.7
131	2.1	2.7	3.4	4.0	4.6
132	2.0	2.7	3.3	3.9	4.5
133	2.0	2.6	3.2	3.8	4.4
134	2.0	2.6	3.2	3.8	4.4
135	2.0	2.6	3.1	3.7	4.3
136	1.9	2.5	3.1	3.6	4.2
137	1.9	2.5	3.0	3.6	4.2
138	1.8	2.4	3.0	3.5	4.1
139	1.8	2.4	2.9	3.5	4.0
140	1.8	2.4	2.8	3.4	4.0
141	1.8	2,3	2.8	3.4	3.9
142	1.7	2.3	2.8	3.3	3.9
143	1.7	2.2	2.7	3.3	3.8
144	1.7	2.2	2.7	3.2	3.8
145	1.6	2.2	2.7	3.2	3.7
146	1.6	2.2	2.6	3.2	3,7
147	1.6	2.1	2.6	3.1	3.6
148	1.6	2.1	2.6	3.1	3.6
149		2.1	2.6	3.0	3.5
150		2.0	2.5	3.0	3.5
151		2,0	2.5	.3.0	3.4
152		2.0	2,5	2.9	3.4
153		2.0	2.4	2.9	3.3
154		2.0	2.4	2.8	3.3
155		1.9	2.4	2.8	3.2
156		1.9	2.3	2.8	3.2
157		1.9	2.3	2.7	3.2
158		1.8	2.3	2.7	3.1
159		1.8	2.2	2.7	3.1
160		1.8	2.2	2.6	3.0
161		1.8	2.2	2.6	3.0
162		1.8	2.2	2.6	3.0
163		1.7	2.2	2.6	2.9
164		1.7	2.1	2.5	2,9
165		1.7	2.1	2.5	2.9
166		1.7	2.1	2.5	2.8
167		1.6	2.1	2.4	2.8
168		1.6	2.0	2.4	2.8
169		1.6	2.0	2.4	2.8
170		1.6	2.0	2.4	2.7

Table 10.10: **Prediction of maximum oxygen uptake (females) from heart rate and work load on a bicycle ergometer.**

Age	Factor	Maximum Heart Rate	Factor
15	1.10	210	1.12
25	1.00	200	1.00
35	0.87	190	0.93
40	0.83	180	0.83
45	0.78	170	0.75
50	0.75	160	0.69
55	0.71	150	0.64
60	0.68		
65	0.65		

These factors are to be used for correction of estimated maximum oxygen uptake:
i) for age differences, or
ii) when the subject's maximum heart rate is known.

Table 10.11: **Correction factors**

Men				
Age	20–29	30–39	40–49	50–59
Poor	Less than 41.9	Less than 35.3	Less than 30.8	Less than 29.4
Fair	42.0–46.3	35.4–38.9	30.9–34.4	29.5–32.8
Average	46.4–51.0	39.0–42,6	34.5–39.2	32.9–36.0
Good	51.1–55.0	42.7–49.9	39.3–44.7	36.1–40.3
Excellent	55.1 or more	50.0 or more	44.8 or more	40.4 or more
Women				
Age	20–29	30–39	40–49	50–59
Poor	Less than 30.0	Less than 26.0	Less than 23.9	Less than 21.0
Fair	30.1–34.9	26.1–29.9	24.0–27.9	21.1–23.9
Average	35.0–39.9	30.0–33.0	28.0–30.9	24.0–28.9
Good	40.0–45.0	33.1–40.9	31.0–37.9	29.0–34.9
Excellent	45.1 or more	41.0 or more	38.0 or more	35.0 or more

Table 10.12: **Maximum oxygen uptake (ml. kg. -1 min -1 STPD) for Australian adults.**

Boys					
Age	Poor	Fair	Average	Good	Excellent
12	←···46.0	46.1–47.8	47.9–51.5	51.6–53.3	53.4 +
13	←···46.0	46.1–47.8	47.9–51.5	51.6–53.3	53.4 +
14	←···46.1	46.2–49.7	49.8–53.4	53.5–55.2	55.3+
15	←···44.8	44.9–48.4	48.5–52.1	52.2–55.7	55.8+
16	←···40.0	40.1–44.8	44.9–49.7	49.8–54.5	54.6+
17	←···34.3	34.4–40.3	40.4–46.4	46.5–52.4	52.5 +
Girls					
Age	Poor	Fair	Average	Good	Excellent
10	←···36.4	36.5–42.4	42.5–48.5	48.6–54.5	54.6+
11	←···36.4	36.5–42.4	42.5–48.5	48.6–54.5	54.6 +
12	←···36.7	36.8–40.7	40.8–44.8	44.9–48.8	48.9 +
13	←···34.2	34.3–37.8	37.9–41.5	41.6–45.1	45.2+
14	←···33.5	33.6–37.5	37.6–41.6	41.7–45.6	45.7 +
15	←···30.1	30.2–34.5	34.6–39.0	39.1–43.4	43.5+
16	←···33.4	33.5–37.0	37.1–40.7	40.8–44.3	44.4 +

Table 10.13: **Maximum oxygen uptake (ml. kg. -1 min -1 STPD) for Australian boys and girls.**

Rating	Men	Women	Boys	Girls
		Exercise Pulse		
Very good	⟵110	⟵116	⟵120	⟵124
Good	100–124	116–130	120–130	124–134
OK	125–140	131–146	131–150	135–154
Poor	141–155	147–160	151–160	155–164
Very poor	⟶155	⟶160	⟶160	⟶165

Table 10.14: **Step test scores.**

Static flexibility measures the range of movement. It does not measure the stiffness or looseness of the same joint during movement.

Dynamic flexibility refers to the ease of movement of joints in the middle of their range of movement.

The Sit-and-Reach test (static flexibility)

The sit-and-reach test is measured with a simple piece of equipment (see Fig. 10.6). If this is not available, a ruler can be placed between the legs with the measure starting at the soles of the feet and moving away from the body.

	Static Flexibility (cm)	
Age	20–39	40–59
Poor	⟵ 1.0	⟵-6.0
Fair	1.1–6.0	-5.9–1.0
Average	6.1 – 10. 0	1.1–7.0
Good	10.1–13.0	7.1–10.0
Excellent	13.1+	10.1+

Table 10.15: **Flexibility classification.**

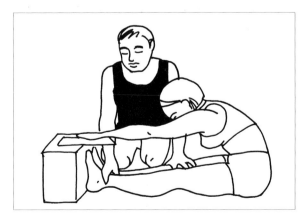

Figure 10.6: **Measuring trunk flexion.**

Procedure

1. This measure should be taken following a total body warm-up. It is best carried out following an aerobic sub-maximal test.
2. The subject sits on the floor with feet on either side of the ruler and pressed against the front board (see Fig. 10.6).
3. Keeping the knees straight, the subject bends at the trunk and gradually pushes the indicator as far forward as possible.
4. Three readings should be taken and the best measure recorded. These can be compared with figures in Table 10.15.

Evaluating Muscular Strength and Endurance

Strength is defined as the ability to carry out work against a resistance. The amount of muscular force which can be exerted against a resistance depends on the size and number of muscles involved; the proportion of muscle fibres engaged in the action; the coordination of the muscle groups; the physical condition of the muscle groups; and the mechanical advantage of the bones employed.

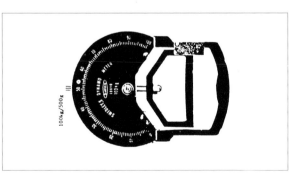

Fig. 10.7: **Smedley's Handgrip Dynamometer.**

	Men		Women	
	Left	Right	Left	Right
Excellent	68	70	37	41
Very good	56	62	34	38
Above average	52	56	30	33
Average	46	50	25	29
Below average	43	48	22	25
Poor	41	45	19	23
Very poor	39	41	18	22

Table 10.16: **Classification of handgrip strength.**

Age:	Sit-ups completed		
Rating	<···29	30–39	40–59
Good	····>17	····>15	····>13
OK	12–17	11–15	10–13
Poor	<····12	<····11	<····10

Table 10.17: **Abdominal strength measure.**

A variety of different techniques are used to measure strength, two of the most convenient being the grip dynamometer test of handgrip strength and the crunch test for abdominal strength and endurance.

Endurance, like strength, can be specific to a particular muscle group. Hence muscular endurance can be measured by a variety of techniques stressing different muscles. One common and relevant measure is that of abdominal muscle endurance, which can be gauged through the 20, 30, 60 or 120 second crunch test.

Measuring handgrip strength

1. The subject holds the dynamometer in one hand, beside by the thigh.
2. The dynamometer is gripped between the fingers and palm at the base of the thumb.

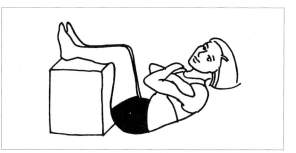

Fig. 10.8: **Measuring abdominal strength**

3. When firmly grasped, it is held away from the body and squeezed vigorously, the subject exerting the maximum force of which he/she is capable.
4. The arm should not be swung or pumped violently. This may increase the recorded score.
5. Two trials should be allowed for each hand, each score being noted. Only the better result counts. Compare with Table 10.16.

Measuring abdominal strength and endurance (see Fig. 10.8)

1. The subject lies on the floor with feet on a standard-height chair so the knees are bent at right angles.
2. Arms are folded in front of the chest, with elbows pointing forward.
3. The subject raises the shoulders off the ground in a 'crunch' position until the elbows touch the thighs. Return then to the position of shoulders flat on the ground
4. Practice should be allowed first.
5. Have the subject carry out as many complete crunches as possible in 20 seconds. If the elbows do not touch the thighs, or the shoulders are not returned to the flat-on-the-ground position, the crunch isn't counted.

THE FITNESS PROFILE

Client Name: Gender: M ❏ F ❏   Date:

Date of Birth: Age: Predicted Max HR: Resting Heart Rate:

BPM: 70–85% of Maximum Heart Rate:

Resting BP: mm/Hg   Weight: Height:

Body Composition

Measurement Protocol

Skinfold Measurements   Site 1   Site 2   Site 3   Site 4

Average of 3 measures:

Sum of sites   Percentage of Body Fat:

Regional Adiposity

Girth Measurements

| Upper Arm: | cm | Chest: | cm | Waist: | cm |
| Abdomen: | cm | Hips: | cm | Thigh: | cm |

Waist-to-Hip Ratio (WHR) Waist cm: Hip cm: WHR:

Flexibility

Sit and Reach Test: Trial One: Trial Two: Sit and Reach Result:

Muscular Endurance

Number of Crunches performed in 20 seconds: Result:

Number of Push-ups performed: Result:

Muscular Strength

1RM - Bench Press: Divided by body weight (   ) =   Rating:

1RM - Leg Press: Divided by body weight (   ) =   Rating:

Assessor's Comments:

Table 10.18: **The Fitness Profile.**

Guidelines for Exercise Testing

- An instructor carrying out sub-maximal testing must be trained by personnel qualified in the protocol being used.

- Tests used must be standardised (preferably with local norm tables). If other tests are devised, these should have readily accessible comparison figures valid and reliable.

- All tests must be carried out to rigid specifications. Attention should be paid in particular to small aspects such as straightening of the knees on a step test, or relaxing a client before a blood pressure measurement.

- All equipment used in testing must be standard and regularly calibrated to the manufacturer's standards.

- If telemetric devices such as EEGs, ECGs or EMGs are used for monitoring, the personnel using such equipment must be fully trained in their use.

- Maximal testing must be carried out to a strictly observed protocol. Oxy-viva equipment must be available. Personnel carrying out the testing must be fully qualified and this testing should only be carried out where emergency medical services can be accessed within 5 minutes.

- All testing must be preceded by a pre-test screen (preferably a written questionnaire). Clients not fulfilling the standards set by this screen (e.g. National Heart Foundation Guidelines, or see Figure 10.1) should then not be tested unless under the supervision of a qualified exercise physiologist or medical practitioner.

- All testing must be clearly monitored by qualified personnel.

- Testing must cease at the client's request.

- Testing should always be followed by a detailed counselling session advising the client of results and, where appropriate, prescribing an individual exercise program to suit the needs of that client.

- If a battery of tests is used, these must be so ordered sequentially that the outcome of each test is not influenced. For example, blood pressure should be taken before sub-maximal testing and after a brief quiet period, such as completing the screening questionnaire.

- Where norms are used, these must be based on a large heterogeneous population and must be up-to-date and preferably (although not always) of local origin.

- Unless specifically aiming to measure one aspect of fitness (e.g. aerobic capacity), testing should involve at least tests of flexibility, aerobic fitness and body composition. Each type of testing should be carried out to protocols laid down in standard texts.

- Body weight/body fat measures must include an assessment of skinfold thickness as well as overall weight. The relevance of this test, as opposed to the use of body weight as a measure of fatness, should be explained to the client in any subsequent counselling session.

- Where a test is intended as a means of medical diagnosis, a medical practitioner must be involved before information is transmitted to the client.

- Clients must be given written information about pre-test requirements such as not eating or not drinking caffeinated drinks before testing. Clients should also be questioned about their immediate exercise efforts to determine whether the effects of any test may be affected by a recent heavy workload.

- If blood is drawn this should be by a qualified person in suitably sterile conditions. Blood should be analysed by a reputable laboratory.

- Adequate warm-up and cool-down procedures must apply for all clients participating in testing. These should be relevant to the specific test to be carried out. For example, flexibility testing should be preceded by stretching to avoid injury to 'cold' muscles and joints.

- All tests must be specific to the purpose. Thus, if increased strength or endurance is an aim of a follow-up program, tests for these should be included.

Nutrition for Active People

The typical Australian diet is high in fat and salt, and low in complex carbohydrate and dietary fibre. It is not suitable for those wanting peak performance in physical activity. It is also not suitable for those who want to minimise their risks of health problems.

No diet, however good, can of itself improve fitness. But a poor diet can certainly decrease the chances of fitness and health. A good diet, like physical activity, is a basic requirement for everyone.

Fitness-oriented people need a diet that is geared much more to health than the typical Australian diet. This does not mean they need to live on grated carrots and sunflower seeds or some strange concoctions of foods. But it does mean they need to make some sensible food choices from the wide range of foods available and so produce a healthier mix of nutrients.

There are important dietary changes fitness-oriented people can make. By manipulating the diet to increase complex carbohydrate, glycogen stores in muscles can be increased to extend muscular endurance. It is also helpful to reduce fats in the diet. This keeps blood fat levels low and helps control the amount of body fat. It also makes sense to decrease the salt and sugar content of the diet and increase dietary fibre. Some of these changes will help athletic performance. All will assist long-term health.

Sports people are a ready target for nutrition quackery. In striving for an edge, many sportspeople take up nutrition-related practices which are useless and sometimes even counter-productive. There's nothing really new in this. The history of sport and physical fitness is riddled with stories of the superior value of particular diets and nutritional supplements. Many of the supplements said to be wonder foods for building muscle or extra energy are worthless; some will actively work against goals of achieving peak performance.

Dietary Guidelines for Australians

Australia has one of the best and most varied food supplies of any country in the world. In spite of such abundance, many people fail to make a healthy selection.

Food group	Main nutrients	Minimum daily amounts
Vegetables, fruits	Vitamin C Vitamin A (as carotene) Fibre Small amounts of many minerals and vitamins	At least 4 servings (1 piece of fruit or 1/2 cup vegetables = 1 serve) Choose a variety, including vitamin C-rich sources such as citrus fruits, tomato, capsicum kiwifruit, rockmelon, strawberries and a dark green or yellow fruit or vegetables for carotene.
Breads, cereals	Thiamin Niacin Protein Some iron Fibre in wholegrain varieties	4 servings or more, depending on energy needs (1 slice bread or small bowl breakfast cereal or 1/2 cup pasta = 1 serve)
Meat, fish, poultry, eggs, dried beans & peas, nuts	Protein Iron Niacin Thiamin Riboflavin	1 serving (1 serve = 75-100g meat or ¼ cup cooked beans)
Milk, cheese, yoghurt (milk can be whole, skim, evaporated or buttermilk	Calcium Protein Riboflavin	Children & adolescents: 600 ml. Adults: 300ml. Pregnancy & lactation: 600 ml (30 g cheese is equivalent to 150 ml milk)
Fats: butter or margarine	Vitamins A and D	15–30 g (1 tablespoon = 20 g)

Table 11.1: **The five food groups.**

Foods that are rich in complex carbohydrate and dietary fibre are often ignored and most people also fail to drink enough water. Such an eating pattern makes it difficult to achieve peak physical performance.

Some people doubt the value of the modern food supply and believe they must rely on pills for nutrients. In fact, Australia has a wonderful selection of healthy foods available and it is perfectly possible to choose an excellent diet. However, there are also many foods that are high in fat, sugar and salt and many with little or no nutritional value. The value of the diet depends on the foods you choose. The idea that the major dietary problem is a lack of vitamins is wrong. Vitamin deficiencies are rare and any diet that is so poor that it lacks vitamins will not be fixed by taking extra vitamins.

Excess weight is common in Australia. It is due to eating and drinking more kilojoules than are needed for metabolism and physical activity (and growth in children). The main culprits for most overweight people are too much fat, sugar and alcohol. Fats and sugar occur in many of our foods and slip down so effortlessly that few people realise the large amounts they are consuming. Foods such as bread, cereals, grains and potatoes are rarely responsible for excess weight. Yet it is these important sources of complex carbohydrate that many people restrict, thus making exercise difficult.

Whether you are lean or overweight, a high fat diet increases the risk of coronary heart disease, high blood pressure, diabetes, gallstones, gout, and breast and bowel cancer. Too much salt increases the chances of high blood pressure, while a lack of dietary fibre upsets the functioning of the intestine and alters the body's chemical balance which controls cholesterol and glucose.

The typical Australian diet has:
- too much fat, particularly saturated fat;
- too little complex carbohydrate;
- too little dietary fibre;
- too much sugar;
- too much salt;
- too much alcohol;
- not enough water;
- too little iron and calcium (mainly in women);
- too much food for our level of physical activity.

The dietary guidelines for Australians seeking to address these major problems are:
- Choose a nutritious diet from a variety of foods (see Table 11.1).
- Control body weight.
- Avoid eating too much fat.
- Avoid eating too much sugar.
- Eat more breads and cereals, preferably wholegrain, and more vegetables and fruits.

- ✗ Limit alcohol consumption.
- ✗ Use less salt.
- ✗ Promote breast-feeding.

Fat

Few people set out to eat a lot of fat but it comes with many of our favourite foods. We are now eating more fat than any previous generation of Australians. The major sources of fat in the Australian diet are as follows:

- 38% comes from oils, margarines and cooking fats (used in fast foods, fried foods, in biscuits, cakes, pastries, snack foods and many processed foods, and spread onto bread, added to vegetables and used in cooking).
- 36% comes from meat (from fatty meats, big steaks and many processed meats as well as the beef fat included in processed foods such as biscuits, pastries and fast foods).
- 15% comes from dairy products (milk, cheese, ice-cream and yoghurt).
- 4% comes from grain foods (hamburger buns, toasted muesli, etc.).
- 3% comes from nuts and peanut butter.
- 2% comes from poultry (mainly the skin).
- 1% comes from eggs.
- 1% comes from seafoods.

To cut down on fat:
- ✗ Choose plenty of low-fat foods such as vegetables, fruits, breads of all types, most cereals and grains and legumes.
- ✗ Avoid fried foods, pastries, biscuits and cakes most of the time.
- ✗ Use minimal quantities of butter, margarine, oil and chocolates.
- ✗ Avoid cream, mayonnaise and oily dressings.
- ✗ Avoid large servings of fatty and processed meats. Choose more seafoods, turkey or chicken (without skin) and look for lean meats such as veal, new fashioned pork, and lean cuts of beef. The leanest part of lamb is the leg.
- ✗ For fast foods, choose sandwiches, salads, toasted sandwiches, a regular hamburger, Lebanese breads filled with salad and hoummus or felafel, char-grilled barbequed chicken (leave the skin) or pizza.

Try to add some fresh fruit.
- ✗ Choose some low fat dairy products such as skim milk, non-fat yoghurt, lower fat cheeses such as cottage, ricotta, Cotto, mozzarella, Swiss or fat-reduced varieties.

Carbohydrates

Energy for fuel can be derived from proteins, fats or carbohydrates. However, carbohydrates are the muscle cells' preferred form of fuel.

Carbohydrates come in two major forms: simple and complex carbohydrates (starches).

Simple carbohydrates (sugar)

The average Australian consumes nearly 1 kg of sugar a week. More than 75% of this is already in foods. A small amount of sugar will not cause problems for most people but the average intake is certainly not 'small'. Sugar has three major disadvantages:

1. Sugar makes fats palatable (you wouldn't eat cakes, pastries, biscuits, chocolates, icecream or desserts if the sugar didn't make the fats taste nice).
2. Sugar has absolutely no vitamins, minerals, dietary fibre, protein or other essential nutrients. It is a useless product from a nutritional point of view.
3. Sugary foods can easily replace other more nutritious foods. For example, many people will eat a sweet or a chocolate bar in place of a more nutritious meal.

Simple carbohydrates include:

Glucose: Mainly formed from the breakdown of all other carbohydrates. Also found in small quantities in fruits, vegetables and honey. (Glucose can also be called dextrose.)

Fructose: The sugar found in fruits and honey (tastes very sweet).

Galactose: A sugar resulting from the digestion of lactose in milk.

Sucrose: Regular cane sugar (made of glucose + fructose).

Lactose: Milk sugar (made of glucose + galactose).

Maltose: Malt sugar from sprouting grains (made of glucose + glucose).

Major sources of sugar include:

- Soft drinks, cordials, fruit juice drinks and other sweetened drinks.
- Confectionery (lollies, chocolates, sweets).
- Biscuits, cakes, pastries.
- Desserts (including icecream).
- Sweetened breakfast cereals (some are nearly half sugar).
- Jams, jellies and spreads.

To cut down on sugar:

- Drink water, pure fruit juices, plain mineral or soda water in place of soft drinks (or use low kilojoule soft drinks).
- Choose fresh fruit for desserts and snacks.
- Avoid large quantities of cakes, pastries and biscuits.
- Gradually give up sugar in tea and coffee.
- Choose fruits canned without syrup.
- Choose unsweetened breakfast cereals such as porridge, weetbix or other wholewheat cereals, puffed wheat or home-made muesli.
- Look for jams without added sugar (avoid those with sorbitol, as this contributes as many kilojoules as sugar).

The term 'sugar' is often only applied to sucrose. You may see food products with the words 'no added sugar' on the label. Check that they don't just contain some other type of sugar. Once in the body, all sugars are eventually converted to glucose.

Complex carbohydrates (starches)

These are molecules made up of thousands of glucose units joined together. They occur in cereals and grains (and foods made from grains such as bread, muffins, pasta and breakfast cereals), vegetables, legumes, nuts and a few fruits (such as bananas and custard apples).

Fruits contain carbohydrate in the form of sugars. In combination with their dietary fibre, we can consider that the carbohydrate in fruits acts like the complex carbohydrates.

Most foods containing complex carbohydrates also contain dietary fibre and a range of minerals and vitamins. Complex carbohydrate should make up 50–60% of the kilojoules in the diet. To increase complex carbohydrate:

- Eat more breads, particularly the wholemeal or wholegrain varieties.
- Eat more cereal products such as oats, wholewheat breakfast products, pasta (preferably wholemeal) and rice (preferably brown).
- Try to include grains such as barley, corn, millet, buckwheat, rye, oats, quick cook wheat and burghul.
- Eat more legumes such as lentils, soya, kidney, black-eye and other beans, chick peas and other types of dried peas.
- Include more vegetables of all types, but especially potatoes.
- Use nuts as a substitute for meat sometimes.

Glycaemic index

It has always been believed that the blood glucose response to carbohydrate was entirely determined by the proportion of simple or complex carbohydrate in the food. Recently there has been a great deal of research to disprove this belief. The glycaemic response (the level, length and rate of increase in blood glucose) of food is not predicted by either the simple or complex molecular structure of carbohydrate, but rather by a variety of factors including fat and fibre content and degree of food processing. The glycaemic index ranks carbohydrate foods on the basis of their rate of appearance in the blood as blood glucose. Carbohydrate that enters the blood stream most quickly has the highest glycaemic index with a ranking of 100, whereas carbohydrate entering the blood stream more slowly will have a lower glycaemic index. There are many applications of the glycaemic index, such as in people with diabetes, those on weight management programs and the enhancement of sporting performance.

Foods with a low glycaemic index rating give a more sustained blood glucose response. These foods are preferable for people with diabetes, and have a role prior to endurance exercise. The consumption of a low glycaemic index meal pre-event (2–4 hours prior to exercise) has shown to prolong endurance exercise capacity. Conversely foods with higher glycaemic index ratings can give a fast burst of carbohydrate, which has been shown to be useful for enhancing the rate of glycogen resynthesis after exercise.

Dietary Fibre

Dietary fibre exists only in plant foods — in grains, breads and cereal products, vegetables, fruits, legumes, seeds and nuts. Animal foods have no dietary fibre. Substances are classed as 'dietary fibre' if the enzymes in the small intestine do not break them down.

Bacteria in the large intestine digest some types of fibre. It is therefore incorrect to say that dietary fibre is not digested. It is simply digested in a different way from other nutrients. During the digestion of dietary fibre, bacteria multiply by the million. Their dead bodies make up more than half the weight of the faeces.

The major types of dietary fibre include:

Pectin: The type of dietary fibre found in apples, citrus peel (and marmalade), jams and fruits.

Cellulose: The 'stringy' fibre in vegetables, also found in grains and cereal foods, fruits, nuts and seeds.

Hemi-cellulose: Actually a number of related substances found in cereals and cereal products (including white bread), vegetables, fruits, nuts and seeds.

Lignin: A 'woody' type of fibre found in cereal husks, root vegetables and pears.

Polysaccharides: Carbohydrate-related substances which occur in foods such as legumes and grains.

Gums: Found in oats and legumes (dried peas and beans).

Saponins: Found in alfalfa, asparagus, chickpeas, eggplant, kidney beans, mung beans, oats, peas, peanuts, soya beans, spinach and sunflower seeds.

Mucilages and gels: Usually added as thickeners in processed foods.

Early measurements of fibre only identified 'crude fibre' which represented cellulose. For this reason, old food tables that list only the crude fibre content of foods grossly underestimate the true dietary fibre content.

The old idea of fibre being 'stringy' does not apply to most types of dietary fibre. Pectin, for example, is a fine white powder which readily absorbs water. The gums in oats also absorb water to form a viscous solution rather than being an obviously coarse fibre. Foods such as celery and lettuce, where you can easily see the strings of fibre, do not contribute much to dietary fibre at all. Other vegetables, legumes and grain products have much more total fibre.

When bacteria in the large intestine are digesting dietary fibre, chemical substances known as volatile fatty acids are produced. These provide nourishment to the cells of the bowel wall. They also control muscular movement of the bowel and may have an anti-cancer effect.

Dietary fibres that are soluble in water (pectin, gums, mucilages) are almost entirely digested by bacteria and produce more of these volatile fatty acids. Rolled oats and legumes are especially useful.

Some types of fibre (gums, mucilages, pectin, saponins) also help control levels of cholesterol and glucose in the blood. They are excellent for sportspeople.

Lignin, a particularly coarse fibre, is hardly digested at all. Cellulose and the hemi-celluloses are digested to a varying extent, depending on your individual intestine and the time food remains in it.

The digestion of various types of fibre also depends on the amount present. If you eat only a small amount of cellulose, for example, most of it is digested. With a higher intake, the bacteria break down less.

The physical condition of some foods is also important. Coarse bran absorbs lots of water and will pass through the large intestine faster than finely ground bran. Coarse bran forms soft faeces; fine bran forms small hard ones.

Populations who eat plenty of dietary fibre have a very low incidence of bowel cancer, diabetes, gallstones, heart disease, diverticular disease, obesity and constipation.

Constipation is a direct result of a diet which is low in fibre (and also lacks sufficient water). However, most of the other conditions mentioned above are likely to be due to several factors, especially a high intake of fat. Foods that are high in dietary fibre are usually low in fat, whereas those that are high in fat generally have little or no dietary fibre. It is therefore difficult to say whether it is the presence of fibre or the absence of fat which provides the greater benefit. It is probably both.

To increase dietary fibre:

- Follow the guidelines for increasing complex carbohydrate.
- Choose wholegrain products wherever possible.
- Eat more fruit.
- Leave skins on fruits and vegetables where practical.

Salt

The salt content of the typical diet is high. Salt is added to processed foods as well as being used in cooking and sprinkled on food at the table. Fast foods are very high in salt (most have much more salt than home-prepared food) and even items you would not think of as being salty, such as cornflakes, have a very high salt content. A bowl of corn flakes has even more salt than a packet of potato crisps.

The taste for salt is learned; by gradually using less salt, the taste buds easily adjust. Once people give up using salt, they usually find salty foods unpleasant.

Some salt is lost in sweat, but the more often you exercise, the less salt is lost. Trained athletes lose very little salt. The more salt you eat, the more water you need to drink. Most sportspeople don't drink enough water at the best of times, and a high salt intake makes any dehydration worse. Long-term, a high salt intake can also contribute to high blood pressure.

To eat less salt:

- Gradually reduce the amount of salt used in cooking until you enjoy the natural flavours of foods without salt. Then reduce salt used at the table.
- Always taste food before adding salt.
- Make greater use of fresh or dried herbs for flavouring foods rather than using salt.
- Choose fresh meats rather than processed meats such as sausages, corned beef, ham, salamis etc. (except for salt-reduced varieties).
- Steam, micro-cook or stir-fry vegetables rather than boiling; the natural flavour will predominate so that you will not need salt.
- Look for unsalted canned vegetables, crackers, butter or margarine, peanut butter and other foods.

Almost all canned foods come in an unsalted version.

- Choose fresh fruit or unsalted nuts or freshly popped corn instead of salty snack items.
- Choose a low salt cereal such as porridge, oats, weetbix, puffed wheat or other packet products which do not have added salt.

Alcohol

Each standard drink contains about the same amount of alcohol. Too much alcohol will adversely affect physical fitness and can damage the liver and brain. One to two drinks a day seem harmless for most people. To cut down on alcohol:

- Drink slowly.
- Have a large glass of water or mineral water before a social occasion so that the first drink is not consumed quickly to quench the thirst.
- Have water or mineral water available at meals.
- Choose low alcohol beer.

Water

Many sportspeople fail to drink sufficient water. Relying on thirst is not enough. After a heavy sweat it can take more than 48 hours for your thirst to tell you to drink enough to replace the losses. A hot climate makes this worse. Alcoholic drinks have a net negative effect on the body's water balance and cannot be considered a substitute for water. At least 6–8 glasses of water a day are needed for sedentary people.

Sportspeople need much more. Weigh yourself before and after a typical training session; the weight loss is water. You can also tell if you are drinking enough water from the colour of your urine. Except for first thing in the morning, it should be almost colourless.

Minerals

Calcium

Calcium is vitally important throughout life. The body maintains the correct level of calcium in the blood for muscle and nerve function by withdrawing or depositing calcium in the bones. A small deficit in calcium intake over the years leads to bones becoming porous, causing osteoporosis.

Changes in female hormones, which accompany menopause, increase the loss of calcium from bones. The greater the calcium content of the bones before menopause, the lower the problem created by hormonal changes. It is therefore important for women to have plenty of calcium for many years before menopause so that the bones can withstand the stress created by ageing.

The recommended daily intake of calcium is 800 mg/day for adults. The best sources of calcium are dairy products (milk — either whole, low fat or skim, yoghurt and cheese). Fish with edible bones (sardines, tuna and salmon), almonds, soya bean milk (fortified with extra calcium) and green vegetables (not spinach) also contain calcium. Sesame seeds are not a very good source, as the oxalic acid they contain forms a chemical complex with calcium making it unavailable to the body.

The amount of calcium retained in bones is decreased by a lack of female hormones (which occurs in women whose body fat level is so low that they do not menstruate), lack of exercise and a diet that is high in protein or salt.

Iron

Iron is part of haemoglobin, which carries oxygen to all body tissues and takes carbon dioxide back to the lungs. In muscles, iron is an important part of myoglobin. It is also essential in the chain of chemical reactions that produce energy in the body.

A lack of iron is common in women because of blood loss every month in menstruation. Early symptoms of iron deficiency include fatigue and irritability. Slimmers are at risk since most popular diets are low in iron. Iron levels can be determined by a blood test.

Men need 5–7 mg of iron a day; women need 12–16 mg — more than twice as much. During pregnancy, requirements are 22–36 mg a day.

Iron is found in oysters, red meats (especially liver and kidneys), poultry, fish, legumes, green leafy vegetables, cereals and wholemeal bread, dried fruits and eggs.

The iron in meat, seafoods and poultry is absorbed best. The iron in wholemeal bread, cereals, vegetables and eggs is absorbed to a lesser extent. Eating even a small amount of meat, fish or poultry will enhance the amount of iron absorbed from vegetables. Vitamin C, found in fruits and vegetables, also increases the absorption of iron, so it makes sense for women to eat a fruit or vegetable at each meal.

Vegetarians can obtain sufficient iron if they eat a variety of legumes, grains, seeds, nuts and vegetables. Those who simply omit most, or all, meat often become iron-deficient.

Iron supplements: It is always best to obtain nutrients from food. However, once you lack iron, supplements are a good way to correct the deficiency.

Supplements which also contain vitamin C will help the iron to be absorbed. Iron supplements should be taken with meals so that the vitamin C from the fruits and vegetables can assist absorption of the iron from the supplement.

Protein and Amino Acids

Most Australians eat plenty of protein. The average sportsperson should aim for 1 gram of protein per kilogram of body weight per day. During weight training, increase this to 1.6 g/kg. Very high levels are not desirable.

Proteins are made up of amino acids. Supplements of amino acids are sold to athletes in the hope that they will have an anabolic effect on muscles. To date, there is no scientifically valid research which shows that amino acids have the claimed effect. Most of the 'results' rely on anecdotal reports, usually from those who are selling the products. A small Australian study looked at the effect of some amino acids on the production of growth hormone (which is thought to stimulate muscle growth). They had no effect. Further scientific studies are required.

Weight Control

It is important that athletes do not carry too much body fat. Body weight itself includes bone, muscle, water and fat. Only an excessive level of body fat is undesirable.

Most slimming diets 'work' by removing water and glycogen from muscles. Many also cause a loss of muscle tissue itself. This makes it difficult to exercise and also leads to future weight gain since it is muscle tissue that burns up kilojoules. When the muscle content of the body is reduced, you may weigh less but you cannot burn up as many kilojoules (muscle burns up lots of kilojoules; fat burns hardly any). Those who try one diet after another find that they need so little food that even a normal food intake increases their body fat.

The misconception that carbohydrates are fattening occurs because popular (but usually unqualified) diet book authors so often recommend low carbohydrate diets. It is the sudden drop in the carbohydrate content of the diet that causes the loss of glycogen and water from the muscles. This appears as a fast loss of weight and makes slimmers believe they are successfully attacking their body fat. However, very little fat loss occurs with these diets; most of the apparent (and temporary) drop in weight comes from a loss of water.

To lose body fat:
* Cut back on all types of fat.
* Avoid alcohol.
* Use little sugar.
* Include enough complex carbohydrate foods to provide glycogen so that you can exercise. Exercise will help remove body fat without losing muscle tissue.

Vitamin Supplements

Most athletes take vitamins. Few need them. If the diet is so poor that vitamins are needed, it will certainly not be providing the right balance of complex carbohydrates and other nutrients. In such cases, taking a supplement will not cure the problem. The way to correct a poor diet is to change the diet!

There is a tendency to believe that 'if a little is good, more must be better'. Some vitamin manufacturers have grown wealthy on that sort of argument.

A deficiency of vitamins (especially the B vitamins) will interfere with performance. That does not mean that extra quantities will enhance performance. It's a bit like the petrol in your car: without it, the car won't go, but if you fill the tank so that it overflows, the car does not go any better than when the tank has just enough petrol. And just as an overflowing petrol tank can be a safety hazard for cars, so can megadoses of vitamins for humans. Enough is enough.

The way to get enough vitamins is to eat plenty of fruits and vegetables, wholemeal bread and other cereal and grain products and to add fish, chicken or lean meat (or a vegetarian alternative).

Megadoses of some of the B complex vitamins can be detrimental to endurance athletes because they deplete glycogen stores faster.

Phony vitamins

Vitamins B_{15}, B_{17}, B-T and P are not true vitamins.

They may sell well and make money for their distributors but they have not been shown to have real benefits for athletes, apart from the belief that they will improve performance.

Other 'miracle' foods such as bee pollen, royal jelly, green magma, zell oxygen, protein powders, herbal supplements, lecithin and orotic acid also have no benefit except for those who believe in their 'magic'.

The Pre-exercise Meal

Most people need to eat about three hours before exercise so they will neither feel hungry nor have a stomach full of food. Choose foods with carbohydrate but little fat such as bread, cereals, fruit, pasta, rice or potatoes. A large fatty meal takes 5–6 hours to be digested and is quite unsuitable.

Avoid sugar or glucose and other high glycaemic index foods in the hour or so before exercise as it can cause a peak in blood sugar, followed by a surge of insulin and a temporary drop in blood sugar level. Weak sugar solutions (about 6–8 per cent) are suitable during endurance events. Once exercise has begun, the exercise itself controls the release of insulin.

Balancing the Diet

The distribution of energy in the typical Australian diet compared with the ideal diet for physically active people is displayed in Table 11.2.

Energy in the diet comes from proteins, fats and carbohydrates (complex and simple). Alcoholic drinks also provide energy from both the alcohol and the sugar they contain.

In order to make an approximate calculation of the percentage of energy coming from each of the nutrients, start by adding up the amount of protein, fat and

Food	Protein	Fat	Carbohydrate
Bread/regular slice	2.0	0.5	15.0
thick slice	3.0	0.8	22.0
roll	5.0	1.0	32.0
Butter 1 tbs		15.5	
Margarine 1 tbs		15.5	
Jam 2 ts			10.0*
Sugar 1 ts			4.0*
Breakfast cereal			
average serve	2.0		23.0(*7.0)
2 Weetbix	4.0		24.0
Muesli 60 g	7.0	5.5	34.0(*13.0)
Toasted muesli 60 g	5.5	10.5	35.0(*15.0)
Milk 200 ml	7.0	8.0	10.0*
Skim milk 200 ml	7.0		10.0*
Flavoured milk 300ml	9.0	9.0	27.0*
Cheese 30 g	8.0	10.0	
Cottage cheese 100 g	18.0	0.5	2.0
Yoghurt 200g	9.0	7.0	12.0*
non-fat 200 g	12.0		14.0*
flavoured 200 g	12.0	7.0	34.0*
Icecream 100 ml	2.0	5.0	11.0*
Fruit/average piece	1.0		18.0*
Beans/e.g. lima	8.0	0.5	23.0*
Fruit juice 250 ml	0.5		30.0*
Vegetables			
salad type	0.5		2.0
cooked (average serve)	1.5		3.0
Peas ½ cup	5.0		12.0
Potato/medium	2.0		18.0
Chips/regular serve	3.0	13.0	20.0
Corn 1 cup	4.5	1.0	26.0
Pasta 1 cup	6.0		50.0
Rice 1 cup	5.0		50.0
Egg 1	6.0		6.0
Bacon 2 strips	8.0	27.0	
Steak T-bone	50.0	46.0	
Lamb chops 2	29.0	40.0	
Sausages 2 thick	22.0	35.0	20.0
Chicken			
1/4 barbecued	24.0	15.0	
Fried, 2 pieces	30.0	29.0	
breast 100 g	25.0	2.0	
Hamburger	31.0	31.0	44.0(*10.0)
Small steak 100 g (no fat)	32.0	7.0	
Pizza/regular	49.0	32.0	89.0
Meat pie	13.0	24.0	31.0
Fish			
grilled fillet (150 g)	27.0	4.0	
battered	21.0	23.0	20.0
Nuts 30 g	5.0	19.0	4.0
Peanut butter, 1 tbs	6.0	10.0	3.0
Oil 1 tbs		19.0	
Cakes			
e.g. date loaf	4.5	7.0	35.0(*26.0)
fruitcake	3.5	9.0	35.0(*28.0)
doughnut	3.0	10.0	18.0(*8.0)
Chocolate biscuit	1.0	5.5	14.0(*12.0)
Ryvita biscuit	1.0		8.0
Rolled oats, raw 30g	4.0	2.0	22.0
Lentils, 1 cup cooked	12.0		24.0

Table 11.4: **Protein, fat and carbohydrate in selected foods.**
NB: Asterisk after carbohydrate means it is a sugar. Sugars and complex carbohydrates contribute an equal number of calories.

	% Cals Current diet	% Cals Ideal diet
Protein	14	10–15
Fat	40	20–30
Complex carbohydrate	15	40–55
Sugars	26	15
Alcohol	5	1

Table 11.2: **Current Australian diet compared with dietary goals.**

carbohydrate eaten, using the figures in Table 11.4. Since every gram of carbohydrate or protein supplies 4 calories, and every gram of fat 9 calories, the percentage of energy coming from each nutrient can be calculated by multiplying:

- the number of grams of protein or carbohydrate by 4;
- the number of grams of fat by 9.

Add total calories and work out the percentage coming from each nutrient. For example, if estimates include 135 grams of protein, 140 grams of fat and 300 grams of carbohydrate, the calculations will be:

Protein	135 g x 4 = 540
Fat	140 g x 9 = 1260
Carbohydrate	300 g x 4 = 1200
Total calories	3000
% Protein	540/3000 x 100 = 18%
% Fat	1260/3000 x 100 = 42%
% Carbohydrate	1200/3000 x 100 = 40%

Alcohol provides 7 calories per gram. A middy of beer has 8 grams of simple carbohydrate and some 11 grams of alcohol. A glass of wine has 0.5 grams of simple carbohydrate and about 12 g of alcohol.

Exercise, Nutrition and Weight Control

Exercise has always been regarded as one of the great linchpins of weight control. Increasing exercise and controlling the amount of food eaten was thought to be the simple way to maintain body weight. By changing the balance between these two factors, i.e. by eating and exercising more or eating less, it was considered there would be an automatic decrease in body weight.

But time and scientific research have taught us that things are never quite as simple as they seem. Although energy balance is obviously important (as the second law of thermodynamics states, energy is neither gained nor lost, it just changes form), a simple physics energy balance formula does not take account of the dynamic nature of the human organism. The human body responds to changes in energy balance, such as a decrease in food intake, by physiological adjustment. It does this by slowing metabolism, changing appetite levels, decreasing the energy cost of effort, and changing body composition in the form of muscle to fat.

For this reason, losses in body fat are resisted. In the case of some people, genetically prone to store fat more readily than others, they are resisted even more strongly than in those with a lesser genetic predisposition. Similarly, it is now known that women, because of their need for energy reserves to get them through pregnancy, resist losses in body fat much more effectively than men. This is done in particular by subtle increases in appetite. A heavily exercising woman may not be aware she is actually eating more as a result of that exercise, but this is often the case, resulting in less weight loss for a given amount of exercise than for a man.

A new approach

The simple energy balance approach to weight loss also doesn't account for other influences on changes in body weight. Biological factors such as genetics and gender, as already discussed are a case in point. Behavioural factors are also important. Early life experiences, such as physical or sexual abuse, particularly in women, can lead to later problems in maintaining a low body weight, which can only be addressed by psychological treatments. Finally, there is the influence of the environment, both the larger, 'macro' environment, which

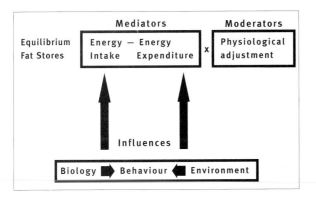

Figure 12.1: **An ecological model for weight control (from Egger and Swinburn, 1996).**

Mediators

All of the effects of the influencing and moderating factors on body fat stores shown in Figure 12.1, are mediated through food and exercise, or more correctly, physical activity.

Energy intake: In recent times, the importance of total calories as a measure of fat-storing energy has been discounted in favour of dietary fat. This is because:

1. Fat is higher in energy (e.g. 9 kcals per gram compared to 4 kcals per gram for carbohydrate and protein.
2. Fat is stored with greater efficiency (i.e. 3% energy loss) than carbohydrate or protein (about 25% energy loss).
3. Fat is non-satiating. It is always easy to eat more in any one sitting.
4. Fat is 'addictive'. We have a craving for fat, which means it is easy to eat more.

From an evolutionary viewpoint it is easy to see why fat is so appealing. For the vast majority of our time on earth, humans have been hunter-gatherers. For a hunter-gatherer it is much more efficient to catch a fatty animal than a lean animal, because this contains more energy and will therefore increase the chances of long-term survival; hence fat, over history, has become attractive to humans. Today however, fat is abundant in processed foods, take-aways and in domesticated farm animals. The most effective way to reduce energy input then is to reduce fat in the diet. It's not necessary, and indeed may be counter-productive, to count calories because this can create a dependency and guilt which only serves to increase fat intake.

The weight loss from this approach is modest and initially may be less than from a conventional low calorie diet. But the longer term results are similar and the reduced-fat, *ad lib* regimen appears to be more acceptable and easier to maintain for most people. All weight loss programs suffer from rebound weight gain, probably due in part to physiological defences against weight loss, but ultimately limited by the high natural settling point of body fat stores for many people living in an 'obesogenic' environment. To keep fat stores below this point often requires considerable effort, which is difficult to maintain over a lifetime.

includes both physical and socio-cultural factors at a national and international level, and the smaller, 'micro' environment, which includes local and personal factors such as the influence of the family, workplace, local weather etc.

This change in thinking about weight has led to a new conceptualisation of the problem. Instead of body weight being regarded as static and influenced purely by food (total calories) taken in and exercise energy (total calories) burned up, all these other factors need to be considered.

A new approach to understanding weight control along these lines has been proposed by Egger and Swinburn (1996) and is shown in Figure 12.1. We'll briefly consider each aspect of this equation here, with particular emphasis on its implications for the Fitness Leader.

Body weight and energy balance

Changes in energy balance occur continuously in humans. Yet these result in comparatively tiny day-to-day changes in body weight. Instabilities of energy balance are usually temporary states restored through appetite mechanisms and/or compensatory physiological adjustments such as changes in metabolic rate or the energy cost of physical activity, as we have seen above. Changes in equilibrium of fat levels may or may not be reflected in changes in body weight, because weight reflects much more than body fat (i.e. it can be bone, muscle or organ weight), although over the long term, changes in weight will reasonably closely reflect changes in body fat.

Energy expenditure: Fat is burned up in the body in response to a number of stimuli. The most important of these is the metabolic rate, which accounts for about 70% of all energy expenditure. Thermogenesis (heat loss) accounts for 15%, and exercise (daily physical activity) for the remaining 15%. As exercise is the most amenable to change, we shall concentrate on this aspect.

The optimum intensity of physical activity for fat burning is controversial. The body utilises carbohydrate or fat as its main energy 'fuels'. Which of these is predominant is dependent on a number of factors, including the intensity and duration of the activity. On the one hand, the proportion of fat utilisation is higher during moderate intensity exercise such as walking, but on the other hand the total amount of energy used is higher during vigorous exercise such as running. It has thus been suggested that vigorous exercise (i.e. around 70–85% of VO_2 max) results in greater absolute fat burning. However, while this may be true for fit people, unfit people tend to burn less fat at all levels of intensity. Obese people generally have low levels of fitness and reduced capacity for fat burning. Therefore, the total amount of vigorous exercise — even if they could carry it out — would not result in as much fat burning in the obese as more moderate intensity exercise which can be sustained for longer periods. The theory and explanation behind this and in relation to general approaches to fat loss is explained in more depth in *The Fat Loss Handbook — A Guide for Professionals* (Egger and Swinburn, 1996).

In practical terms, the emphasis for weight loss in obese people should therefore be on regular, low-to-moderate intensity recreational and 'incidental' physical activity. This is also in line with recent evidence verifying the use of low-moderate intensity activity for metabolic fitness (primarily improvements in blood pressure, blood fats and blood sugars). The promotion of high intensity exercise for the obese may also be counterproductive because it could be expected to be uncomfortable, and could only be sustained for a short duration. Exercise can be 'planned', in the sense of an organised activity regime, or made up of increased 'incidental' exercise. And while the former is probably necessary to ensure an appropriate amount of activity for fat loss, the latter is often all that is needed, at least in the early stages of any fat loss program in the very obese and usually immobile.

Moderators

Physiological adjustment: Physiological adjustment refers to the metabolic, and in some cases, behavioural changes that follow a disequilibrium in fat or energy balance and which prevent excessive fluctuations in body weight. For example, the response to a negative fat or energy balance may initially be increases in appetite or decreases in physical activity, followed by weight loss; declines in the rate of fat burning and resting metabolic rate then occur until a new fat and energy balance is achieved. Physiological adjustment may be more or less vigorous, depending on biological factors such as gender, age or genetic makeup.

One of the implications of physiological adjustment is that frequent 'plateaus', or slowing of weight losses with time, may represent normal physiological opposition to energy disequilibrium. Hence the graph in Figure 12.2 shows the expected real decline in body weight with a weight loss program in contrast to a straight line theoretical loss which is often promoted by weight loss programs. In Figure 12.2 it can also be seen that those who have been overweight for a long time are likely to have longer plateaus and shorter drops off these plateaus than those who have only been overweight for a short period.

Physiological adjustments could be expected to be more vigorous in response to weight loss than weight gain, especially in lean individuals, and it is possible that they may also be more vigorous following rapid changes than with slow changes. Hence, there is a greater need to concentrate on long-term goals for reducing equilibrium fat levels, rather than short-term

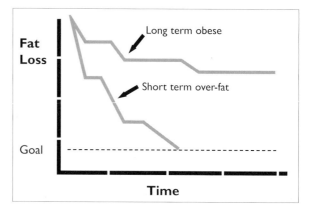

Figure 12.2: **Plateaus in weight loss caused by physiological adjustment.**

— and usually temporary — weight loss. This questions the ethics of fitness programs that advertise large weight losses in a short period.

Influences

The model of weight control shown above explicitly includes extra- and intra-individual factors affecting energy balance; in particular, environmental, biological and behavioural influences. Each of these needs to be considered in detail in any valid weight control program.

Environmental influences: The environment contains a multitude of changing factors which affect obesity, many of which occur simultaneously. In 1995, a group of Australian scientists graded the 'modernity' of six Papua-New Guinea villages based on indices such as the use of technology, education levels, occupation and housing. The level of modernity correlated closely with the mean body mass index of the inhaitants of each village, with levels of physical activity appearing to be the most important factor affecting this. This suggests that we are getting fatter in the western world largely because we now have machines to do all the physical work for us that was done using person-power in the past.

The complexity of environmental factors can be broadly categorised into 'macro'-environment (affecting the whole population) and 'micro'-environment (affecting individuals). In general terms the macro-environment determines the prevalence of obesity in a population and the micro-environment, along with biological and behavioural influences, determines the presence of obesity in an individual. Macro- and micro-environmental settings can have either a physical or socio-cultural basis.

Environmental influences represent the public health arm of the obesity problem. While the macro-environment remains non-supportive, programs aimed at influencing behaviour at the individual level can be expected to have only a limited effect. Historically, epidemics are only controlled once environmental factors are included in the paradigm and subsequent public health action occurs. Examples of this are infectious diseases (draining swamps for malaria), road crashes (median barriers, traffic islands for pedestrians) and smoking (taxation, smoke-free legislation). In a similar fashion, no significant reductions in population levels of obesity seem likely until attention is given to modifying the environments that facilitate its development. The Fitness Leader cannot expect to have a big impact on the macro-environment, but can exert a major influence on the micro-environment. The micro-environment can be influenced by checking on food supplies in an individual's house, the availability of labour-saving devices, access to exercise equipment, the use of vehicles for transport instead of walking. Environmental 'audits' in fact need to become a significant part of the Fitness Leader's armament.

Biological influences: Biological factors known to influence body fat levels include age, gender, race, hormonal factors (such as puberty, pregnancy and menopause) and a wide range of genetic factors. Heritability accounts for about 25–40% of the variance of body mass index, suggesting that obesity has a strong genetic base, and given the wide genetic influences on physiology and behaviour, it is very likely to be polygenic. i.e. to have many genes influencing the problem. There are significant sex differences in energy balance and fat storage, particularly during the female reproductive years. The differences between the sexes are apparent early in life, become greatest with the onset of puberty, then tend to decrease with the changes in female hormone status in post-menopausal women. Fat loss and maintenance of lower equilibrium fat stores also becomes more difficult with age. Finally, there is increasing evidence of racial differences in the rate at which individuals gain and lose fat.

Behavioural influences: The traditional behavioural influences in obesity development are popularly characterised as 'sloth and gluttony'. They imply a potential for wilful control over the major forces producing obesity. Biological and environmental influences are not determined by the will of the individual, and even in behaviour willpower is only part of the picture. Behaviours are the result of complex psychological factors, including habits, emotions, attitudes, beliefs and cognitions developed through a background of learning history. Habits are learned ways of responding which tend to resist change. Cognitive processes involve patterns of thinking. Emotions represent the affective state of consciousness, while attitudes and beliefs reflect dispositions and accepted opinions with regard to a person or thing. A common example of interactions between these factors is the vicious cycle of failure, guilt, depression, lowered self worth and counter-productive habits which result from and lead to repeated failures with weight loss diets. Although there is no evidence to suggest that psychopathology is a major cause of obesity, these individual psychological factors have to be considered as having both a cause and effect association. Interventions designed to deal with these psychological factors at an individual level are a vital part of any overall strategy.

Summary

1. Physical activity should be regarded as vital to the long-term maintenance of fat loss.
2. The primary recommended form of physical activity for fat loss and long-term maintenance of fat loss is long, low-to-medium intensity, gentle aerobic exercise.
3. It is not necessary for physical activity to be continuous in order to achieve fat loss. An overall increase in day-to-day physical activity through 'planned' and 'incidental' activity should be encouraged.
4. The appropriate level of intensity of physical activity for fat loss with optimal safety in someone who is fat and unfit is low–moderate (i.e. 40–60% VO$_2$max)
5. Intensity of physical activity may be extended with increasing fat loss and fitness, and this should be prescribed by a relevant medical or exercise specialist.
6. Physical activity in the early stages of a program is perhaps best based on distance covered in the case of walking, cycling, swimming, etc. With increasing fitness, heart rate and then perceived rate of exertion (PRE) can be used to determine the intensity of physical activity.
7. Non weight-bearing activities such as cycling, swimming or rowing should be given less support in fat loss programs, except where clients may need this initially for comfort or motivation.
8. Anaerobic activity should never be prescribed for fat loss, particularly in cases where fitness levels and medical contraindications are unknown.
9. Any physical activity program for fat loss should be accompanied by a reduction of fat in the diet.
10. Special problems of big people — such as chapped thighs caused by walking — should be recognised and accommodated for by appropriate recommendations (such as the wearing of lycra shorts in the case of chapped thighs).

Guidelines for Exercise for Weight Control

Research into weight control and obesity in recent years shows that i) not everyone gains or loses body fat at the same rate, ii) that counting calories, both in food and in exercise, is insufficient.

Fat in foods is regarded as the prime culprit on the input side of the equation and every effort should be made to help clients reduce their dietary fat intake by providing detailed education about where fats are hidden in foods and the alternatives that can be eaten.

Exercise for fat loss is now clearly regarded as being different from exercise for fitness. Instead of high intensity, long duration activity at an elevated heart rate, any increase in movement is seen as important for fat loss. Two types in particular are recommended: planned movement, such as a regular exercise program, and 'incidental' activity, such as that gained through effort otherwise expended by machines or another person.

Special Problems and Exercise Instruction

Most exercise theory is based on the principle that the exerciser is 'normal'. Yet surveys show that up to 80% of the population suffer one or more forms of disability, ranging from minor respiratory ailments to paraplegia.

Many normal conditions such as pregnancy and advanced age, as well as common health disorders, can be adversely affected by poorly prescribed exercise. Therefore it is essential for Fitness Leaders to understand and follow basic safety parameters for managing these individuals during exercise.

The following exercise guidelines provide the basis for safe exercise prescription for people with a variety of special needs. It is important to note that as a Fitness Leader you are not qualified to make medical assumptions with respect to people with conditions that require specialised medical advice and/or treatment. Rather, the role of the Fitness Leader is to work in conjunction with other health professionals such as doctors, physiotherapists, etc. in an effort to provide safe and effective exercise programs.

More severe types of disability usually require individualised, specialist attention. However, when working with any large population the Fitness Leader will encounter people with common conditions that command special consideration when prescribing exercise.

Allergies to Exercise

Allergic reactions to exercise were relatively unheard of in the past. But with increased participation in structured exercise, reports of exercise-related allergies are becoming more common.

Symptoms

Exercise-related allergies can be classified under three headings:
1. Exercise-induced anaphylaxis (allergic 'shock')
2. Exercise-related forms of urticaria ('nettlerash')
3. Exercise-induced asthma.

Most common symptoms of points 1 and 2 are pruritis (itchiness), skin rashes and swelling; these are common in people who are involved in sustained vigorous activities, especially runners. In severe cases, anaphylaxis may be life-threatening, such as with allergies to bee stings, penicillin, etc. Other symptoms can include heart-beat irregularities, stomach and nervous system upset, repeated coughing and lowered blood pressure.

Symptoms usually begin about 5 minutes after starting to exercise, but might not occur until after it is over; also, they don't necessarily occur after every exercise session. Generally the reactions subside after 30 minutes to 4 hours, but headaches can last several days in some cases.

Causes

The causes, in most cases, aren't known. But the reaction is more common in individuals who are generally allergic, together with those with a family tendency to exercise-induced allergy.

Asthma is common in about 10% of the population (see below) but with proper medication it can be well controlled. However, allergists point out that exercise-induced asthma can also occur in otherwise non-asthmatic individuals as a result of a reaction to certain food or drugs taken before exercise: aspirin, for example can lead to severe shortness of breath and wheezing. It is not known how common this reaction is.

Tips for the Fitness Leader

Where an obvious reaction to exercise occurs, Fitness Leaders should look for a 'pattern' in the preceding 12–24 hours. Headaches after morning exercise where only coffee is taken beforehand, for example, implicate coffee (or perhaps an ingredient of coffee such as caffeine) directly as the culprit. In other cases, an allergy to a particular type of solid food (e.g. shellfish, cheese, celery, etc.) may also show up after vigorous exercise. In less common cases, any food eaten within 2 hours of exercise can cause a reaction.

Outdoors, allergies to grasses or pollens can become more severe with exercise, and these can even have cross-reactions with certain foods or drinks.

In indoor exercise classes, there might be allergic reaction to dust on carpeted floors. Cross-reactions are also possible here, but these are not yet clearly understood.

Food allergies can be systematically and safely checked by eliminating either the suspected food from the diet, or re-introducing foods one at a time after a 24-hour fast. If this is not successful, an allergist should be consulted. Medication may be necessary. In severe cases where cause can't be found and there's no reaction to medication, the only option might be to modify the type or duration of the exercise program.

Anorexia

Anorexia is a condition characterised by severe under-weight and an obsession by the sufferer to remain extremely thin. This is generally effected by self-starvation in combination with obsessive exercise behaviour.

The condition is most common in women under 30 and seems to be caused by a psychological problem resulting from a struggle to establish a sense of control and identity. As most sufferers come from a comfortable middle-class background, parental relationships seem to play some part in the problem.

Symptoms

Anorexia is characterised by weight loss, ammenorhoea (cessation of periods), and other effects of starvation including reduction in metabolic rate, body temperature, pulse and blood pressure and an increase in anaemia and sleep disturbances. People with anorexia typically don't see themselves as abnormally thin, but take pleasure in extreme weight loss. They won't admit hunger and often develop bizarre eating habits such as avoiding foods believed to be 'fattening', not eating at all for long periods, or eating only a limited range of foods. Diuretics and laxatives are often used to reduce body fluids and weight, and if the anorexic does occasionally give in to eating binges, this is compensated for by self-induced vomiting.

A major consideration for the Fitness Leader is that, because of their enthusiasm and denial of their condition, it's often difficult to convince people with anorexia that extreme exercise is not advisable.

Tips for the Fitness Leader

Individuals more than 20% under ideal weight should be advised to get medical approval before starting an exercise program.

In many cases, people with anorexia are unaware that they are dangerously underweight. This often needs to be pointed out in a firm manner, and the possible hazards explained. However, as one of the main characteristics of the disease is denial of the problem, the subject has to be approached cautiously.

Anorexia is a psychological infirmity. Correction requires extended and expert treatment, which is available in most major hospitals. The role of the Fitness Leader should be to act as a point of first contact rather than as an immediate source of treatment or advice.

Anorexia is unlikely to be as widespread a problem as obesity in affluent societies. Nevertheless, some experts believe it may exist in up to 1% of adolescent girls, making it common enough to warrant attention by Fitness Leaders.

Arthritis

Although it takes many forms, arthritis is basically an inflammation around the joints. The causes are varied and not well understood, and treatments are primarily symptom-oriented. The symptoms are pain and loss of movement, followed by swelling and a change in the shape of the joint.

Rheumatoid arthritis is more common among the 20–55 age group, and women are three times more likely to suffer from it than men. Osteoarthritis occurs as part of the ageing process. It happens mainly in weight-bearing joints (hips, knees and spine) and can be associated with previous injury.

Although exercise is likely to help the arthritic patient in increasing mobility as well as in improving general health, it should never be thought that excessive exercise will overcome the problem. Prescription should include regular stretching and strengthening exercises, with a progression to more dynamic aerobic activities once pain has begun to subside. Sometimes the exercise effect can be assisted by pain-relieving heat or cold therapy, or through stretching within the comfort of a heated pool. Stretching can progress from static to active-assisted to active as improvement occurs.

Strengthening exercises can help reduce the effects of immobilisation of a joint. Isometric exercises in the early stages are probably best, with isotonic activities being introduced as the symptoms of the disease begin to improve.

People with arthritis can also benefit from aerobic exercise, but fatigue and increased stress on an affected joint should be avoided. For this reason, weight-supported exercises such as swimming and cycling are preferable to jogging for long-term improvements. Most experts agree that although jogging does not predispose to arthritis in the healthy individual, it is probable that repetitive jarring on hard pavements will accelerate damage in the arthritic joints of the lower limbs. Since increased temperature is a good indication of inflammation, the golden rule of thumb with arthritic clients is 'Train cold joints, rest hot joints'.

Tips for the Fitness Leader

For people with arthritis, exercise capacity is often limited by joint function rather than cardiovascular function. Therefore, exercise should be programmed to accommodate patterns of stiffness and pain.

During exercise, people with arthritis should tolerate only mild discomfort. Prescribe extended warm-ups and cool-downs with low-to-moderate intensity conditioning bouts. Encourage weight-supported activities like aquarobics, swimming, stationary cycling, etc. The mode of exercise prescribed is dependent upon the joints that are affected

Encourage individuals to perform all exercises through full range of movement, while controlling the speed of movement. Avoid activities that require sudden jarring movements; if necessary, encourage use of aids (eg. a chair) to provide support and stability.

Asthma

Asthma is a breathing disorder caused by constriction of the air ducts in the lungs. It generally runs in families and results from an over-sensitivity of the mucous membrane lining and muscles of air ducts. The air ducts react to specific irritants such as house dust, pollens, animals, nervous tension, or smog and fumes. In most cases, asthma is also brought on by vigorous exercise. It was once thought that the majority of children with asthma would grow out of it, but research has shown that up to 50% can be still symptomatic at adulthood.

The exact causes of asthma are not known. However, it is now suspected that changes in the sensitivity of the air ducts are caused by moisture losses in the airways related to ventilation and cooling. For this reason it's thought that asthmatics will react more adversely to exercise in dry conditions.

Asthma is a chronic condition that, when managed well, can allow participation in most activities; however, its severity does vary considerably. Modern medications have made exercise possible for many asthma sufferers. Bronchodilators such as Ventolin can help prevent asthma episodes that were previously triggered by exercise.

With continuous and graded exercise, people with asthma can develop greater respiratory muscle tone, which can lead to a decreased need for medication. Cardiovascular exercise is the preferred option for this group; resistance training exercises such as bench press and pullovers can be prescribed to help strengthen the respiratory muscles.

Tips for the Fitness Leader

Care should be taken to ensure an adequate and gradual warm-up, particularly in cold conditions. Because winter air is coldest (and therefore usually driest) in the early morning, people with asthma may find exercising easier on winter afternoons. If possible encourage the client to take up swimming or water exercises, where inhaled air is warm and moist. In general encourage exercise in warm, moist environments, (e.g. swimming, warm aerobic floors, etc.).

Be sensitive to the fact that up to ⅓ of children in an exercise program may show some symptoms of asthma (e.g. coughing heavily after exercise). This should be acted on by reducing the exercise load and seeking medical advice.

Encourage those with chronic wheezing or coughing after exercise to get medical attention. Medication may reverse the effects, but lack of medication can lead to chronic lung damage.

Avoid exercises that necessitate lying on dusty floors or carpets, which could contain allergenic substances like house dust, animal hair, etc.

If individuals are on prescribed medication, use them prophylactically. Advise the client to take oral medication before and, if necessary, during an exercise session. If this doesn't give relief the exercise should be discontinued.

Encourage regular monitoring of peak flows to help identify days when exercise may be contraindiacted.

Exercise Anaemia

In general, the scientific literature leans away from advocating vitamin and mineral supplements for athletes and heavy exercisers provided that they eat a varied and balanced diet.

But one issue on which advice is more divided is that of iron. Are there possible deficiencies of iron in endurance athletes (particularly women and adolescents), and will iron supplements help?

The function of iron

Iron ('haem') is contained in a protein molecule ('globin') called haemoglobin, which exists in red blood cells in the bloodstream. Protein and iron combine like a motorcycle and sidecar. Without the sidecar an extra passenger couldn't be transported: without iron, the globin couldn't carry oxygen to the working muscles of the body because iron is needed to bind oxygen chemically.

A decrease in haemoglobin in the bloodstream can lead to low oxygen utilisation, resulting in constant tiredness and low energy. The condition is called 'anaemia', which simply means 'lack of blood'. The anaemic person can generally be identified by paleness around the mouth, whiteness of the blood vessels of the eyes, and a pervasive feeling of tiredness.

There is also an indication that heavy exercise may decrease haemoglobin levels in some people because of either:

1. An increase in total blood volume occurring with endurance exercise, which isn't matched by an increase in haemoglobin.
2. Reduced haemoglobin production resulting from low iron stores. Although the reason for the low iron observed in some athletes (e.g. runners) isn't known, it could be through:
   - low iron in the diet;
   - low absorption of iron in the digestive tract;
   - high rates of iron loss.
3. A breakdown of the red blood cells (which carry haemoglobin) through physical trauma.

Although some surveys of athletes have shown haemoglobin levels around the lower level of what's regarded as the normal range (i.e. 15 g/100 ml), there's little indication that this would cause problems. Unless they have an extremely poor diet, it's unlikely that iron levels in most exercisers should cause any concern. Two possible exceptions to this are heavily exercising women (particularly vegetarians who have had children) and highly active adolescents, who may be on poor and hence low iron diets.

The problem may be exaggerated in women because of heavy blood (and hence haemoglobin) losses in menstruation, and in adolescents because of extra iron needed during the growth spurt.

Tips for the Fitness Leader

If anaemia is suspected in an exerciser, he/she should be referred for a blood test, and medical advice if necessary. Women in the at-risk category should be advised to have a blood test at least annually.

Iron poisoning is possible (although unlikely with the doses recommended in most supplements), hence iron supplements without medical advice are never advisable. In any case, studies have shown that supplements don't significantly increase haemoglobin in those with normal levels.

Individuals at risk or suspected of anaemia can be advised to eat a diet high in iron, protein, vitamin B_{12} and vitamin C. Good foods in these categories are leafy vegetables and organ meats like liver and kidney. Vegetarians may need a vitamin B_{12} supplement.

Because vitamin C helps the absorption of iron, foods high in both vitamin C and iron (leafy vegetables and citrus fruits) should be encouraged.

Diabetes

Diabetes is a chronic disease that is hyperglycaemic in nature; that is, it causes unusually high blood sugar (glucose) levels. Diabetes is a complex medical disorder that exists in two forms. Type I (insulin-dependent or juvenile onset) diabetes which generally occurs in young people and is related to a deficiency of the pancreas in producing insulin. The other, Type II (non-insulin dependent or mature onset diabetes), generally begins later in life and is due to an insufficiency of insulin action; this condition is closely related to central obesity.

Insulin acts as a bridge allowing the transport of glucose from the blood into body tissues. Because the diabetic's supply of insulin is impeded, blood glucose levels remain high or fluctuate rapidly, and body cells are 'starved' of energy. If an individual's diabetes is not controlled he/she may easily tire, feel weak, and experience rapid weight loss. Other symptoms of diabetes are polyclipsia (thirst), polyphagia (incessant hunger) and polyuria (frequent urination).

In most cases of juvenile onset diabetes, regular daily insulin injections are required to balance blood sugar levels, but in adult onset cases dietary management is usually sufficient. In some cases where insulin is used, it is possible to misjudge the balance between insulin dose and physical activity, which results in hypoglycaemia (low blood glucose). This can cause light-headedness, lack of judgment, fainting and even death if continued for long enough. In these cases the simple ingestion of food with a high glycaemic index rating usually offers a quick reversal to the situation.

The control of diabetes generally involves five steps: 1) diet, 2) exercise, 3) managing body fat levels, 4) insulin, and 5) oral hypoglycaemics. Diabetes affects about 3% of the Australian adult population, but the incidence of the disease is rapidly rising, to the extent that estimates suggest that up to 5% of the adult population could be sufferers by the turn of the century. There are two possible reasons for this. Firstly, there is an increasing proportion of aged in the population and type II diabetes is to a degree age-related. Secondly, medical advances have meant that diabetics can now survive to reproduction age where they might not have in the past, therefore — because the disease is inheritable — more diabetics (or potential diabetics) are being born.

In terms of management, it is now accepted that regular aerobic exercise has a positive effect on the body's sensitivity to insulin (the hormone that allows glucose to be used as fuel). By maintaining a regular exercise program, people with diabetes can reduce their chances of suffering many of the vascular complications associated with diabetes.

Although the mechanism is not fully understood, regular exercise can decrease insulin requirements, sometimes by as much as 50%. This can be of enormous benefit because of the possible harmful effects of long-term insulin therapy. For some people with Type II diabetes who need to use insulin, starting an exercise program may reduce or even replace the need for extra insulin. Hence, exercise is a key component of the long-term treatment of diabetes.

Finally, aerobic exercise aids in the treatment of obesity and overweight, which is a major cause of diabetes. In fact, it is estimated that about half of all people with diabetes in affluent societies could be 'cured' by the reversal of obesity to normal weight — and staying that way.

If insulin and/or food intakes are not regulated during exercise, the main risk for people with diabetes is hypoglycaemia. Therefore, exercise, food and insulin regulation should be carefully considered by a person with professional expertise in diabetes management.

In undiagnosed or poorly controlled cases of diabetes, exercise may be contraindicated. It could have the opposite effect to that outlined above and cause further hyperglycaemia, which can result in keto-acidosis and ketotic coma. The signs of this are a dry tongue, hyperventilation (long, deep, sighing breaths), rapid and weak pulse, intense thirst and frequent urination, constipation, muscle cramps and altered vision. Hyperglycaemia is less common with exercise and can only be treated with insulin injection. If there is confusion, the subject should be treated for hypoglycaemia and a doctor called immediately.

Tips for the Fitness Leader

When diabetes is well controlled and the individual has no other medically based contraindications, there are no exercise restrictions. However, recent research suggests that insulin sensitivity is greatest in 'slow twitch' muscle fibre. Hence exercise utilising slow twitch fibres (i.e. aerobic exercise) will have the most benefit for stable management.

Regardless of this, a medical screen should be performed and advice on insulin and dietary changes should be sought. Clinics for the treatment of diabetes are now available in most major city hospitals. For further information, regular contact should be made with these. All people with diabetes should be screened for cardiovascular complications, which may contraindicate exercise, i.e. high blood pressure, heart rate abnormalities, etc.

As exercise increases the rate of insulin absorption in muscles, it is wise for the diabetic on insulin not to inject at an area being used most for exercise — particularly the leg. Abdominal walls or the arm can be used as the site of injection for exercise such as running.

Prescribe gradual increases in exercise intensity to avoid possible cardiac arrhythmias.

Encourage blood glucose monitoring and postpone exercise until 60 to 90 minutes after insulin injection, or until late in the insulin activity period. In general, avoid erratic timetabling.

Always have some form of glucose readily available for the treatment of possible hypoglycaemic reactions to exercise or over-insulinisation; 15–30 grams of readily absorbed carbohydrate every 20–30 minutes.

People with diabetes should not exercise alone; they should inform someone of their condition if exercising in a new environment.

Hypertension

Hypertension is a medical condition indicating abnormally high blood pressure. It is known as the symptomless disease, because it's often the cause rather than the outcome of complications. Traditionally, it has been treated with anti-hypertensive drugs, but some side effects of these have led practitioners to look to more natural forms of treatment.

The questions for the practitioners are: Does exercise lower blood pressure? If so, in what form should it be taken, and with what precautions, by hypertensive people?

Exercise and hypertension

Regular aerobic exercise has been thought to help decrease blood pressure through either:
- chronic dilation of the arteries;
- chronic reduction in heart rate and increase in stroke volume resulting in the heart working less hard to supply blood to the working muscles;
- reduction in body weight, which has consistently been shown to lower blood pressure.

The value of exercise in helping to relieve hypertension is not wholly clear, but many studies have shown reductions in people with moderate/borderline hypertension.

However, those diagnosed with higher than moderate hypertension generally need to combine drug and healthy lifestyle therapy.

Given the limitations of the research, it has to be concluded that there's not enough scientific evidence yet to suggest that exercise could be substituted for medication as a treatment for hypertension. However, the greater the improvement in aerobic capacity (VO_2 max) after an exercise program, the more the expected reduction in blood pressure.

Changes in blood pressure noticed after an extended exercise program seem to be independent of body weight; it's not known, however, if this is independent of changes in fat as distinct from weight. Although it seems that exercise may be beneficial for the hypertensive person, precautions should be taken.

Tips for the Fitness Leader

Consult the client's doctor before prescribing a full exercise program, preferably one who can monitor blood pressure responses during a sub-maximal stress test.

Prescribe an exercise program which is aerobic in nature with extended warm-ups and cool-downs and low-to-moderate intensity conditioning bouts.

Avoid isometric exercises, inversion treatments and sudden changes in temperature (sauna baths to cold showers, etc.) as these can increase blood pressure and put extra strain on a weak heart.

Don't use pulse rate as a measure of exercise intensity. If blood pressure medications are being used that affect the normal heart rate response to exercise, use the perceived rate of exertion (PRE) scale. In addition, review regularly any antihypertensive medications once the exercise program has begun.

Look for the occurrence of bradycardia (slowing of HR by more than 10 bpm) with no changes in exercise load. If this occurs, seek medical advice.

During resistance training avoid maximal lifts, performing the valsalva manoeuvre, and high intensity isometric contractions.

Reduce load when performing lifting exercises above shoulders, or prescribe another exercise in preference. Wherever possible, reduce exercises involving large amounts of muscle mass, e.g. use single leg press in place of a double leg press or squat.

The Senior Client

As ageing occurs the objectives of exercise programs change. For example, in young adults increases in aerobic capacity or muscular strength may be desired. However, maintenance of physical independence and bone strength become a greater priority as people age. Although ageing is an inevitable and normal part of life, there are certain physiological limitations that occur with age which must be considered when designing exercise programs for seniors. These are:

- Basal metabolic rate decreases by approximately 2% per decade after age 20 years. This is thought to be due to atrophy of fast twitch muscle fibres, which also leads to reductions in absolute strength.
- Reductions in joint mobility can occur as a result of arthritis and/or reductions in the elastic properties of muscles and tendons.
- Cardiorespitatory changes occur, such as decreases in resting and maximal heart rates, VO_2 max and lung capacity.
- Reductions in bone density, strength and mass occur — more common in women.
- Reduced co-ordination and slower reflexes.

Tips for the Fitness Leader

Promote increases in overall daily activity, avoid jarring, sudden changes in posture and begin with moderate activities such as walking, cycling or aquatic exercise.

Perform extended warm-ups and cool-downs and encourage flexibility exercise post warm-up and conditioning bout.

If any of the following have occurred, exercise may be contraindicated or at least require specialist advice:

- severe angina or previous cardiac infarction;
- congestive cardiac failure;
- uncontrolled hypertension
- uncontrolled cardiac arrhythmias;
- recent deep vein thrombosis.

Children

It is important to note that children are not little adults. Children are anatomically, physiologically and psychologically immature, therefore special precautions are needed when they participate in exercise. A child's cardiovascular system is much less efficient then an adult's, children demonstrate higher heart rates, smaller stroke volume and lower blood pressure. In addition to cardiovascular differences children also demonstrate musculoskeletal differences. Some of the differences between adults and children are:

Children overheat very easily. They generate more heat at a given exercise intensity; they don't perceive that they are hot; they sweat less and they sweat later. In addition, they don't conduct, radiate or convect heat as well as adults, due to lower peripheral circulation.

Although children are good at rehydrating at home, where palatable drinks are usually readily available, they often forget to replace fluids during exercise. During exercise children should be encouraged to consume 100–150ml of fluid every 15–30 minutes.

Children generally have less body fat and get cold more quickly.

Children do not like high intensity activities; they are much less tolerant of lactic acid than adults. The least suitable form of exercise for children is high intensity exercise lasting for 20–90 seconds. Children prefer short-term intermittent activities with a recreational component.

Because the bones of children are relatively immature, overall they are much softer and have a greater propensity to fracture. They are especially prone to greenstick fractures. In addition, because of immature hence soft epiphyseal growth plates, children are predisposed to epiphyseal damage, which increases the chances of joint and bone malalignment.

Children are more likely than adults to suffer repetitive strain type injuries. The most frequent problem in this area is inflammation of the epiphyseal regions. This commonly occurs through repetitive overloading of tendons.

The Cardiac Client

This group includes those individuals who have diagnosed coronary artery disease (they may have a history of angina but have not yet had a cardiac event), who have experienced one or more heart attacks (generally referred to as post-MI or myocardial infarction patients), and those who have had some form of cardiac surgery such as angioplasty or bypass. Exercise prescription for this group is usually prepared under the supervision of a post-cardiac care specialist. However, the Fitness Leader can play an important long-term support role.

Tips for the Fitness Leader

Prescribe an exercise program that is aerobic in nature with extended warm-ups and cool-downs and low-to-moderate intensity conditioning bouts.

Become familiar with heart rate responses to any medications that clients are taking.

If angina is experienced at an exercise session, it is recommended that the individual should note the intensity at which it was experienced and keep their intensity level below that point at the next exercise session. If angina is experienced at two or more exercise sessions, all exercise should cease until the individual has consulted his/her physician.

Avoid isometric exercises, inversion treatments and sudden changes in temperature (sauna baths to cold showers, etc.) as these can increase blood pressure and put extra strain on a weak heart.

Don't use pulse rate as a measure of exercise intensity if blood pressure medications are being used that affect the normal heart rate response to exercise — use the perceived rate of exertion (PRE) scale.

Look for the occurrence of bradycardia (slowing of HR by more than 10 bpm) with no changes in exercise load. If this occurs, seek medical advice.

During resistance training avoid maximal lifts, performing the valsalva manoeuvre and high intensity isometric contractions.

Choose exercises carefully for post-bypass patients — some exercises may cause discomfort, i.e. pec deck or lying dumbbell flyes.

Exercise and Pregnancy

Original guidelines for exercising during pregnancy were published in 1985 by the American College of Obstetricians and Gynecologists (ACOG). Since then ACOG have released updated guidelines. It is important to note that ACOG did not countermand the original guidelines as a result of the update, hence many of the original guidelines of 1985 still stand. Encouraging pregnant exercisers to follow guidelines for appropriate frequency, intensity, duration and type of exercise during gestation is crucial for the safety of both the mother and the developing fetus.

When exercise is contraindicated

Exercise during pregnancy is ideal for women who are considered by their doctor to be at low risk and who were exercising before pregnancy. However, pregnancy is not the time to start an exercise program for the previously unfit. ACOG has published a list of contraindications to exercise, which should be discussed with all pregnant women who wish to exercise.

Contraindications to exercise during pregnancy can be broken into two categories; absolute and relative.

Absolute contraindications are conditions in which exercise is not recommended during pregnancy. They are:

- history of three or more spontaneous miscarriages;
- ruptured membranes;
- premature labour;
- diagnosed multiple pregnancies e.g. twins;
- intrauterine growth retardation (baby size is smaller than expected);
- incompetent cervix (cervix becomes softer and more open than normal);
- placenta praevia (portion of the placenta sits over cervix making it vulnerable to detachment);
- pregnancy-induced hypertension;
- venous thrombosis or pulmonary embolism (clots to legs or lungs);
- known cardiac valve disease;
- primary pulmonary hypertension;
- maternal heart disease.

Relative contraindications are conditions which must be reviewed by an obstetrician, who will make the decision as to whether exercise should be undertaken.

- Hypertension
- Anaemia
- Thyroid disease
- Diabetes
- Extremely over- or underweight
- Extremely sedentary
- Breech presentation in third trimester
- History of bleeding during pregnancy

Screening during pregnancy: All pregnant exercisers should be appropriately screened and have their doctor's permission to exercise, preferably in writing. Because there are specific screening questions which apply to pregnant exercisers, a separate screening questionnaire should be added to the standard health screen. It should include the absolute or relative list of contraindications and consider issues such as:

- Overall activity level.
- Daily activities (ie. if she is on her feet all day, recommend non-weight bearing exercise).
- Sporting involvements (sports involving potential for falling and contact sports are contraindicated during pregnancy).
- Record of previous injury (ligament laxity during pregnancy may make her susceptible to reinjury, shin pain can become aggravated because of increased weight, etc.).

Effects of Exercise on the Fetus

Primary considerations are the acute effects of exercise on the fetal temperature, heart rate, and oxygenation as well as its chronic effects on gestation and birthweight. Because the mother has greater exercise tolerance than the fetus, any exercise program should be designed with the wellbeing of the developing baby as the prime consideration.

Fetal temperature

Overheating of the fetus can have serious effects, particularly in the first trimester, when the incidence of miscarriage is highest and birth defects are most likely to occur. If the mother overheats during exercise, the fetus will be hotter than the mother because it cannot dissipate heat effectively. ACOG guidelines state that the maternal core temperature should not exceed 38°C.

To avoid overheating, the mother should understand that her core temperature is related to both the intensity and duration of exercise and that it is therefore important to avoid both prolonged and high-intensity exercise. Recommendations for staying cool include:

- staying well-hydrated, (use the 'water-bottle pact' — make a deal with each pregnant exerciser that she will drink an entire water bottle's contents during her workout);
- avoiding exercise on hot, humid days;
- wearing light, loose-fitting clothing, using fans during hot weather, and avoiding saunas and steam baths.

Do not be lulled into a false sense of security if a pregnant woman is not sweating. Core temperature starts to rise before perspiration occurs.

Blood flow to the baby

Exercising in the supine position (on the back) may also affect blood flow to the baby. In this position, the enlarging uterus can compress the vena cava (a large vein that carries blood back to the heart), thereby decreasing the amount of blood that returns to the heart and reducing cardiac output. This can result in a reduction in blood flow to the fetus and to the mother's head, causing dizziness or light-headedness. The ACOG recommends that no exercise be done in the supine position after week 16. However, there is evidence that range of movement, low intensity, supine exercise does not adversely effect cardiac output until after week 35. Fitness Leaders should be conservative when using the supine position with a pregnant exerciser. Do not allow her to lie on her back for prolonged periods of time (2–3 minutes is maximum) or to perform rapid or vigorous movements, and always advise her to be aware of the signs of reduced cardiac output such as dizziness or light-headed feelings. If these occur, she should immediately roll onto her left side and then slowly sit up.

Fetal heart rate

A change in fetal heart rate suggests that a change has occurred in the fetal environment. Marked decreases in fetal heart rate in response to exercise may indicate fetal distress (such as a lack of oxygen or overheating). One study showed that fetal heart rates were normal as long as the exercise intensity stayed moderate (around 140 bpm). However, when intensity increased to an average maternal heart rate of 180 bpm, fetal heart rate decreased significantly in 20% of the participants. This drop in fetal heart rate occurred during the first 3 minutes of the recovery phase and lasted 1–10 minutes. The implications of this are:

- that strenuous exercise above 140 bpm should be avoided.
- that the cool-down phase of a workout should be gradual, since fetal risk may be greatest immediately after the conditioning bout of a workout.

Birthweight and gestation

The most marked increase in fetal weight occurs in the third trimester. Intense exercise at this stage can result in decreased birthweight and/or a shorter than normal gestation period. These are not considered healthy birth outcomes. One study followed pregnant joggers and aerobics participants who attended 3 to 11 high intensity exercise sessions per week (the average heart rate was 166 bpm). The birthweights were lower in exercising mothers, particularly in the babies of the mothers who continued to exercise more than 4 times per week after week 28.

It is not known which specific combinations of frequency, duration and intensity are likely to cause problems. Current ACOG guidelines state that exercise intensity should not raise the maternal heart rate above 140 bpm, and duration should not exceed 15 minutes. However, preliminary results of other studies suggest these parameters may change to 150 bpm for maternal heart rate and possibly 25 minutes for exercise duration.

Pregnant exercisers should check with their doctor to ensure that maternal weight gain and the fetal growth are increasing at a satisfactory rate throughout the pregnancy. If not, their exercise may need to be curtailed and their nutritional intake assessed.

Maintaining a recommended target heart rate

Fitness Leaders should encourage pregnant exercisers to be realistic about exercising in moderation. Some women may need to be discouraged from trying to keep up with non-pregnant exercisers or compete with what they were able to do prior to pregnancy.

Pregnant women should be taught how to measure their heart rate and check it regularly, preferably at 5–10 minute intervals, during exercise. Alternatively, some fitness centres may have heart rate monitors that pregnant women can borrow. While monitoring heart rate is crucial when exercising during pregnancy, the use of Borg's perceived rate of exertion scale should not be used alone because it tends to underestimate heart rate responses in pregnant women. Also, advise pregnant women that an increase in the resting heart rate is a normal physiological response and does not reflect a decrease in fitness. It is not abnormal for a resting heart rate of 70 bpm to be as high as 100 bpm by the end of a pregnancy.

Another effective strategy for getting pregnant exercisers to stay within a safe level of exercise is to provide an Information Handout which outlines the rationale for the guidelines, namely protection of the fetus, and provides suggestions for exercise. For example, to decrease intensity, pregnant exercisers should be encouraged to change from an intermediate or advanced aerobics program to a lighter pace program, or to modify higher impact movements to lower impact movements (i.e. from running to marching). In some fitness centres, stationary bicycles are placed close to the aerobics floor so that pregnant participants can cycle rather than run or do complicated movement patterns in exercise classes.

Effects of Exercise on the Mother

Pregnancy-related changes that influence exercise performance

As the body shape changes during pregnancy, so does the centre of gravity, which affects stability, balance and co-ordination. Consequently, exercise classes that involve rapid directional changes, lots of turns and twists and quick move changes, may put the pregnant exercisers at risk of injury.

The hormone relaxin is increased in the body during pregnancy. This hormone increases joint laxity, which may make the pregnant exerciser more susceptible to injury. For this reason, stretching should be done very gently.

Exercise-related discomforts

An important consideration with pregnant exercisers is the amount and type of discomfort they may feel when exercising. Many experience urinary frequency and incontinence, breast tenderness, back pain and general fatigue. Exercises such as push-ups, tricep dips, exercises performed in the kneeling position and arm exercises that go across the chest might feel uncomfortable. Kneeling on-all-fours may cause wrist stress due to increased weight. When in the prone (lying on the front) position, the mother may have the feeling that she is 'squashing' her baby.

Whilst the discomforts experienced by pregnant exercisers are usually minor, they merit care and attention from the Fitness Leader. You should be aware of these and help your pregnant participants to develop an exercise program or selection of classes to attend that minimises their risk of injury and discomfort. Low-impact classes are often more comfortable than high-impact classes. Fitness Leaders should provide alternatives to 'problem' exercises and suggest strategies for handling segments in classes which may cause problems (such as what to do during abdominal tracks where too much time may be spent lying on the back).

Separation of the rectus abdominus

Another concern for the pregnant exerciser is the separation of the rectus abdominus at the linea alba (the strip of connective tissue that joins the abdominal muscles in the centre). This occurs in about 30% of pregnant women and is not normally accompanied by pain. Pregnant women who want to continue doing abdominal work should ask their doctor to check for separation between the abdominal muscles at each antenatal visit.

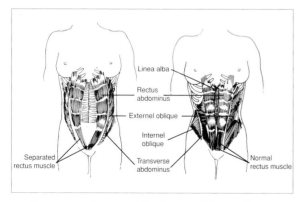

Figure 14.1: **Rectus abdominus and linea alba.**

If separation does occur, abdominal exercises should cease. It is recommended that the muscle be supported or braced by crossing the hands over the abdominal area when doing any crunch-type movement.

Pelvic floor strengthening

Kegel exercises (those used to strengthen the pelvic floor muscles) should be performed during pregnancy. There are two ways to increase the strength of the pelvic floor muscles. One is a long, controlled isometric contraction of these muscles. The other is a short, hard, contract-release contraction. Both types of exercises should be done. Sets of 5-10 contractions performed several times each day should be prescribed. Strong pelvic floor muscles will recover more quickly and be stronger after delivery and be helpful in preventing urinary incontinence. Women with serious incontinence problems should be referred to a qualified physiotherapist who specialises in pelvic floor conditioning.

Benefits of water-based exercise

Compared with the same workload on land, exercise in the water can decrease the mother's heart rate by up to 10 beats per minute and cause fetal heart rate changes to be less marked. Because water conducts heat 25% faster than air, the woman's core temperature will not rise as quickly and her fetus will have an extra cushion of protection against overheating. Because water supports body weight, problems with balance and co-ordination are eliminated. The pressure of the water also decreases the venous pooling effect, helping to reduce the effects of swelling during pregnancy. The mother's prone body position (when swimming freestyle and breaststroke) also promotes optimal blood flow to the fetus. All of these things combine to make water-based exercises one of the best forms of exercise during pregnancy.

When to Stop Exercising

Finally, make sure that you, as the Fitness Leader, and your pregnant exercisers are aware of the signals to STOP EXERCISE. If at any time during an exercise session, the woman feels very hot, faint, dizzy, short of breath, experiences vaginal bleeding, has palpitations, blurred vision, disorientation, severe or continuous headaches, lower abdominal pain, tightness or cramping, back pain or pubic pain they should stop immediately and consult their obstetrician.

Legal aspects of exercise during pregnancy

If the outcome of a pregnancy is not a normal, healthy baby, the chances are the parents may try to place blame on any aspect of the pregnancy that could have caused the problem. If a pregnant woman under your care trips or falls, causing her to have pregnancy or baby-related problems, you could be held responsible. It is critical that you have the appropriate Fitness Leader certification and current professional indemnity insurance. Make sure pregnant exercisers are properly screened and have a doctor's permission to exercise. Try to avoid the attitude that it is too hard to give pregnant exercisers special care and attention.

Use the 'Exercise During Pregnancy Fact Sheet' as a guide to help educate your pregnant clients about safe exercise during pregnancy.

Conclusion

Exercise during pregnancy can be a healthy, safe, beneficial experience if care and caution are applied and Fitness Leaders and pregnant women are knowledgeable.

There are many benefits of regular moderate exercise during pregnancy, including improved cardio-respiratory fitness, improved muscle strength and tone, increased self-esteem, increased sense of wellbeing, feeling in control of your body and its changing shape, heightened body awareness and weight control. Pregnant mums need special care from their Fitness Leaders, who should always strive to keep up-to-date on the issues related to exercise and pregnancy.

Exercise During Pregnancy — Fact Sheet

The information contained in the following 'Exercise During Pregnancy Fact Sheet' is copyright. If reproduced in any form the following acknowledgement must appear clearly on the document. 'This work is copyright and has been reproduced with the permission of its authors — Lisa Champion, MSc. (Exercise Science) and Dr. Maureen O'Neill, BBS., Grad.Dip.Ex.Rehab., FRACP.'

Exercise during your pregnancy can be a very beneficial experience if you are conscious of the precautions to take and knowledgeable about the effects that exercise can have on you and your developing baby. The guidelines and limitations for exercise should start as soon as you know you are pregnant, or begin trying to become pregnant. If you have any specific questions or concerns, please ask your Fitness Leader or obstetrician.

1. Understand that the limitations put on exercise frequency, intensity and time are for the benefit of the developing baby, not for the mother. Normally, the mother can handle exercise much better than the baby.

2. Avoid overheating. Your growing baby does not have the same ability to dissipate heat as you do. Consequently, if you get overheated when you are exercising, the baby may be put at risk. This is especially true during the first trimester, when the most important growth, cell reproduction and formation is occurring. To avoid overheating:

a) Avoid prolonged exercise. Limit the more strenuous phase of your aerobic exercise to 15 minutes or less. Give yourself breaks during the workout to rest and cool-off.

b) Stay well hydrated. Drink plenty of water before, during and after your workout. Take a water bottle with you, and make a deal with yourself to drink its entire contents by the end of the workout.

c) Do not use sweating as an indicator of how hot you may be getting. Your core temperature may rise without any accompanying perspiration.

d) Avoid exercising on hot, humid days. Use fans during hot weather.

e) Wear light, loose-fitting clothing. Cotton is best.

f) Avoid saunas and steam baths at all times during pregnancy. Your core temperature may be rising without an associated feeling of being hot.

3. Avoid high intensity exercise. Studies have indicated that when a mother's heart rate stays in a range of approximately 140 bpm, the fetus has no abnormal responses. However, when maternal heart rate averaged 180 bpm, indications of fetal distress were present. This strongly suggests that high intensity exercise needs to be avoided. To keep exercise intensity at a safe level, follow these guidelines:

a) Change from an intermediate or advanced aerobics program to a lighter pace program. Modify the level of impact (do mainly low-impact movements) and use less vigorous arm movements. You may have to modify your program more if you are exercising in a weight-bearing mode (aerobics, jogging, using a stair-climbing machine, etc.) than if you are exercising in a non-weight bearing mode (swimming, cycling.) This is because your increased weight will add to the overload effect of the exercise.

b) Learn how to measure your heart rate, and check it regularly. For a ten-second-exercise heart rate check, it should be 23 beats or less. If it is higher, lower the intensity and re-check in five minutes to assure that you are not working too hard.

c) Be realistic about the need to exercise in moderation. You do not need to keep up with non-pregnant participants or compete with what you were able to do before pregnancy.

d) Have a prolonged cool-down after the aerobic portion of your workout. Stopping exercise suddenly, or going directly from aerobic exercise to lying on the floor can also have detrimental effects on the fetus. Gradually reduce the intensity of the aerobic phase of your workout and, after you have finished, get a drink, move around and cool off before commencing floor exercises or stretching.

4. Avoid frequent and prolonged exercise after week 28 of your pregnancy. Even with moderate exercise intensity, frequent (more than four times per week) exercise after week 28 has been associated with decreased birth-

weight and gestation duration.

5. An increase in your resting heart rate is a normal response to pregnancy. If your normal resting heart rate is around 70 bpm, it can go as high as 100 bpm at rest by the end of your pregnancy. This is a completely normal physiological change and should not be taken as a sign that you are becoming less fit.

6. Limit the amount of exercise that you do lying on your back. This is of particular concern from your second trimester on. Exercising on your back (as when doing abdominal exercises) could cause a reduction of blood flow to your heart and head, causing you to feel faint and lightheaded. More importantly, the blood flow to the placenta and baby can decrease. Limit the amount of time on your back to 2–3 minutes and if you begin to feel at all dizzy or lightheaded, turn onto your left side and rest.

7. About 30% of pregnant women will experience a separation of the rectus abdominus during pregnancy. If this does occur, abdominal exercises should cease. Even if it is not a problem, it is recommended that you support your abdominal muscle by crossing your hands over the abdominal area (bracing) when doing any crunch-type movements. Do not do full sit-ups at any time. If you continue to do crunches when pregnant, your obstetrician should regularly check the separation of your abdominal muscle. If separation or discomfort occurs, stop doing abdominal exercises. In addition, all exercises performed in the supine position should be avoided.

8. Avoid the use of handweights over .5 kg in weight. Heavier weights have been shown to increase the heart rate higher than 140 bpm. New Body exercise classes with no weights could be a perfect alternative to a normal aerobics class. The use of hand weights should be avoided if pins and needles are being experienced in your hands.

9. The only form of resistance training that should be done during pregnancy is low weight, high repetition work with an emphasis on endurance rather than strength training. Avoid heavy strength training during your pregnancy.

10. Perform Kegel Exercises. These exercises are useful for strengthening the pelvic floor muscles, aiding in your recovery from labour and delivery and helping to avoid stress incontinence. While seated or lying down, pretend that you are trying to stop yourself from urinating. The small muscles you are squeezing are your pelvic floor muscles. Hold each contraction for 10–15 seconds and repeat at least ten times. If stress incontinence is a problem for you, do this several times each day and see a qualified physiotherapist who specialises in pelvic floor conditioning.

11. Wear a good, supportive bra. This helps to provide support for your enlarging and possibly tender breasts.

12. Avoid rapid changes in direction. As your body shape changes, so does your centre of gravity which may effect your stability, balance and co-ordination. Exercise classes that involve rapid directional changes, lots of turns and twists and quick move changes may put you at risk of injury. Either avoid them, or modify the exercises to make them simpler and less complicated.

13. Be very cautious if you are doing Step exercise classes. For the same reasons as above, you may be at risk of injury or falling when stepping. From the first trimester, lower the step height — preferably working on a platform only. Do not use handweights, do not perform propulsions, and do not participate in complicated Step classes. In the second and third trimester, or at the time that you begin to show, Step classes are not recommended because the changes in your body may effect your balance. Step classes should only be done by experienced pregnant exercisers and if so, with extreme caution. If you have never done Step classes, do not begin them during pregnancy.

14. PUMP™ classes. These classes should be approached with caution. If you have not previously participated in PUMP classes don't begin during pregnancy. Experienced PUMP exercisers should be very cautious as some of the exercises may cause back, knee or other joint pain.

15. Stretch gently. The hormone relaxin is increased in your body during pregnancy. This hormone causes increased joint laxity, which may make you more susceptible to injury. Be cautious and gentle with your stretching.

16. With exercise, pregnant women sometimes experience low blood sugar levels, resulting in lightheadedness or faintness. A light snack approximately 2 hours before exercise should prevent this. Carry a small carton of fruit juice to your workout in case this occurs.

17. STOP EXERCISE! If at any time during your exercise session you feel very hot, faint, dizzy, short of breath, experience vaginal bleeding, have palpitations, blurred vision, disorientation, or severe or continuous headaches, STOP IMMEDIATELY. It is also important to stop if you experience lower abdominal pain, tightness or cramping, back pain or pubic pain. If you experience any of these symptoms, consult your obstetrician.

References

Alter M.J. (1996) *Science of Flexibility*. Human Kinetics, Champaign Illinois.

Baechle T.R. (1994) *Essentials of Strength Training and Conditioning*. Human Kinetics, Champaign Illinois.

Batman P. and Van Capelle M. (1995) *The Exercise Guide to Resistance Training*. FIT4U Publications. Australia.

Brooks G.A. and Fahey T.D. (1984) *Exercise Physiology. Human Bioenergetics and its Appliactions*. Macmillan Publishing Company, New York.

Clark N. (1997) *Nancy Clark's Sports Nutrition Guidebook*. Second Edition. Human Kinetics, Champaign Illinois.

de Vries H.A. (1986) *Physiology of Exercise for Physical Education and Athletics*. WCB Group, USA.

Donnelly J.E. (1990) *Living Anatomy*. Second Edition. Human Kinetics, Champaign Illinois.

Egger G. and Swinburn B. (1996) *The Fat Loss Handbook — A Guide for Professionals*. Allan & Unwin, Sydney.

Fleck S.J. and Kraemer W.J. (1997) *Designing Resistance Training Programs*. Second Edition. Human Kinetics, Champaign Illinois.

Heyward V.H. (1991) *Advanced Fitness Assessment & Exercise Prescription*. Second Edition. Human Kinetics, Champaign Illinois.

Howley E.T. and Franks B.D. (1997) *Health Fitness Instructor's Handbook*. Third Edition. Human Kinetics, Champaign Illinois.

Lindle J. (1995) *Aquatic Fitness Professional Manual*. Aquatic Exercise Association, Florida.

McCardle W.D., Katch F.I. and Katch V.L. (1996) *Exercise Physiology — Energy, Nutrition, and Human Performance*. Fourth Edition. Williams and Wilkins, Baltimore.

Miller P.D. (1995) *Fitness Programming and Physical Disability*. Human Kinetics, Champaign Illinois.

Pyke F.S. (1991) *Better Coaching — Advanced Coach's Manual*. Australian Coaching Council.

Stanton R. (1994) *Eating for Peak Performance*, Allen & Unwin. Sydney.

Thompson C.W. and R.T. Floyd (1994) *Manual of Structural Kinesiology*. Twelfth Edition. Human Kinetics, Champaign Illinois.

Van Gelder N. and Marks S. (1987) *Aerobic Dance-Exercise Instructor Manual*. International-Dance Exercise Association (IDEA) Foundation, California.

Wilmore J.H. and Costill D.L. (1994) *Physiology of Sport and Exercise*. Human Kinetics, Champaign Illinois.

Index

Federation for International Sport, Aerobics and Fitness

FISAF is an international, independent, democratic, non-profit organisation

which is the largest confederation of fitness industry organisations in the world.

FISAF members form a synergistic network of expertise, resources and activities.

The scope of activity of FISAF and its members includes the following: instructor training

and certification, development and production of professional resources, publication of industry

journals, staging of conventions, expos and sport aerobic championships.

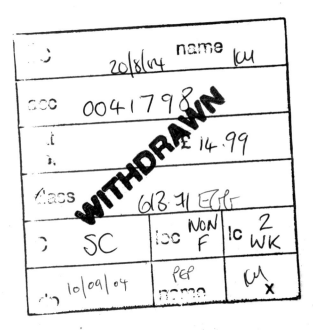